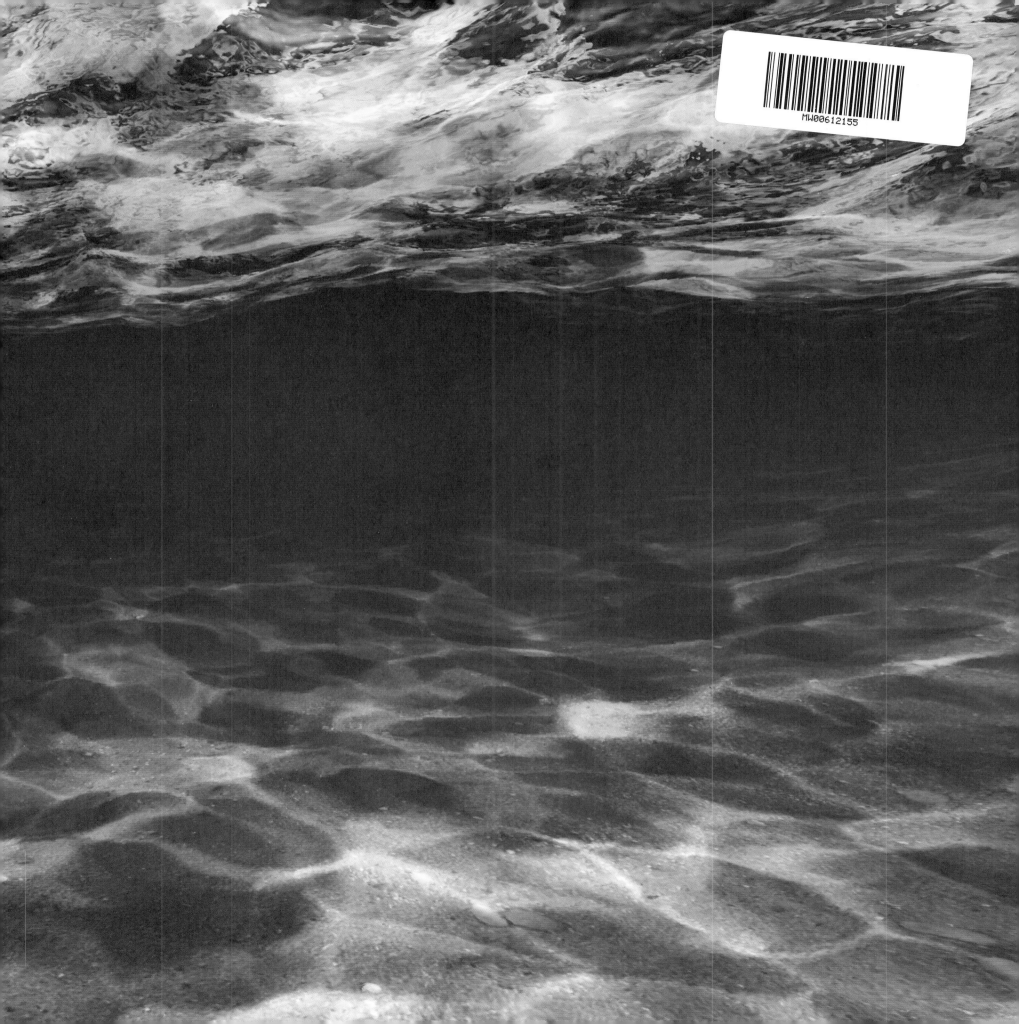

PROJƎCT YOU

A lifestyle guide to true health and longevity

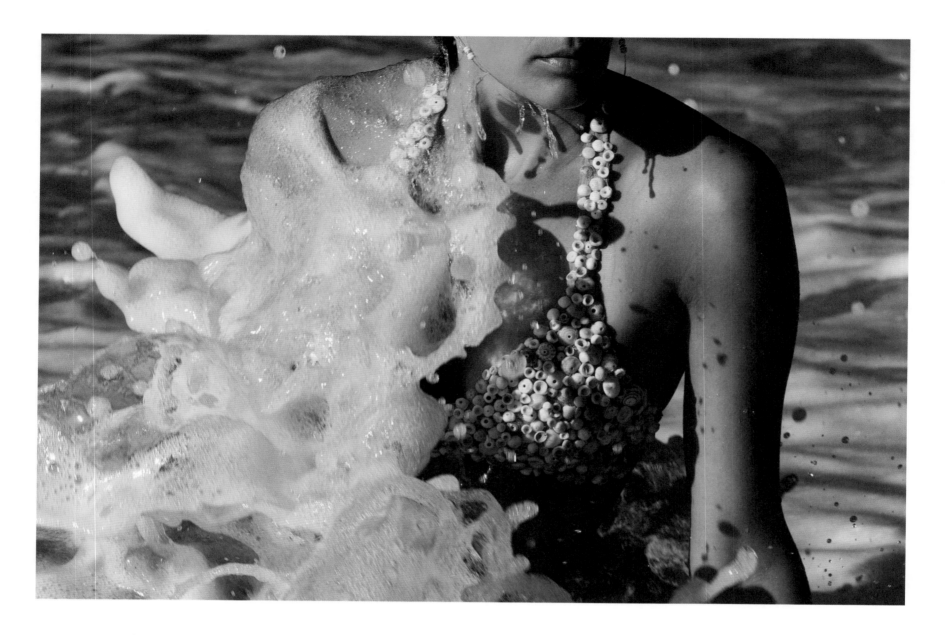

Library of Congress Cataloging-in-Publication Data

First designed, printed and published December 2017
Project You: A lifestyle guide to true health & longevity
ISBN - 978-0-6481677-4-7

Smudge Culinary Travel Publishers

PROJECT YOU

A lifestyle guide to true health and longevity

WRITTEN BY
Neely Mack

EDITOR
Samantha Walravens

PHOTOGRAPHY
Franck Berthuot – Creative Director of Photography
Brydie Mack
Maria Simon
Tim McKenna
Lauren Ross
Maria Teresa Bravo
Dean Bentley
Brooke Lydecker
Russel Rainbow
Caroline Woodham

DESIGN
Hilary Andersen

"If there is magic on the planet, it is contained in water."

Loren Eiseley

MISSION STATEMENT

My goal is to help you achieve true health and longevity by engaging the three pillars of wellness — internal (nutrition and gut health), physical (exercise and sleep) and emotional and spiritual self-care — that together will help your body act and feel younger.

ABOUT THE AUTHOR

Neely Mack is a health and wellness advocate, founder and CEO of a fashion accessories company, and mother of twins. A former competitive athlete, Neely began a lifelong search for "true health" after suffering debilitating health problems in college, where she played tennis at a high level. She has spent the past 20 years traveling the world, researching the healing properties of "superfoods" that slow down or reverse the aging process, and studying supercentenarian cultures where people live to ages well beyond 100 years.

She invites you to join her in her journey to true health and wellness.

Learn more at *projectyoubewell.com*

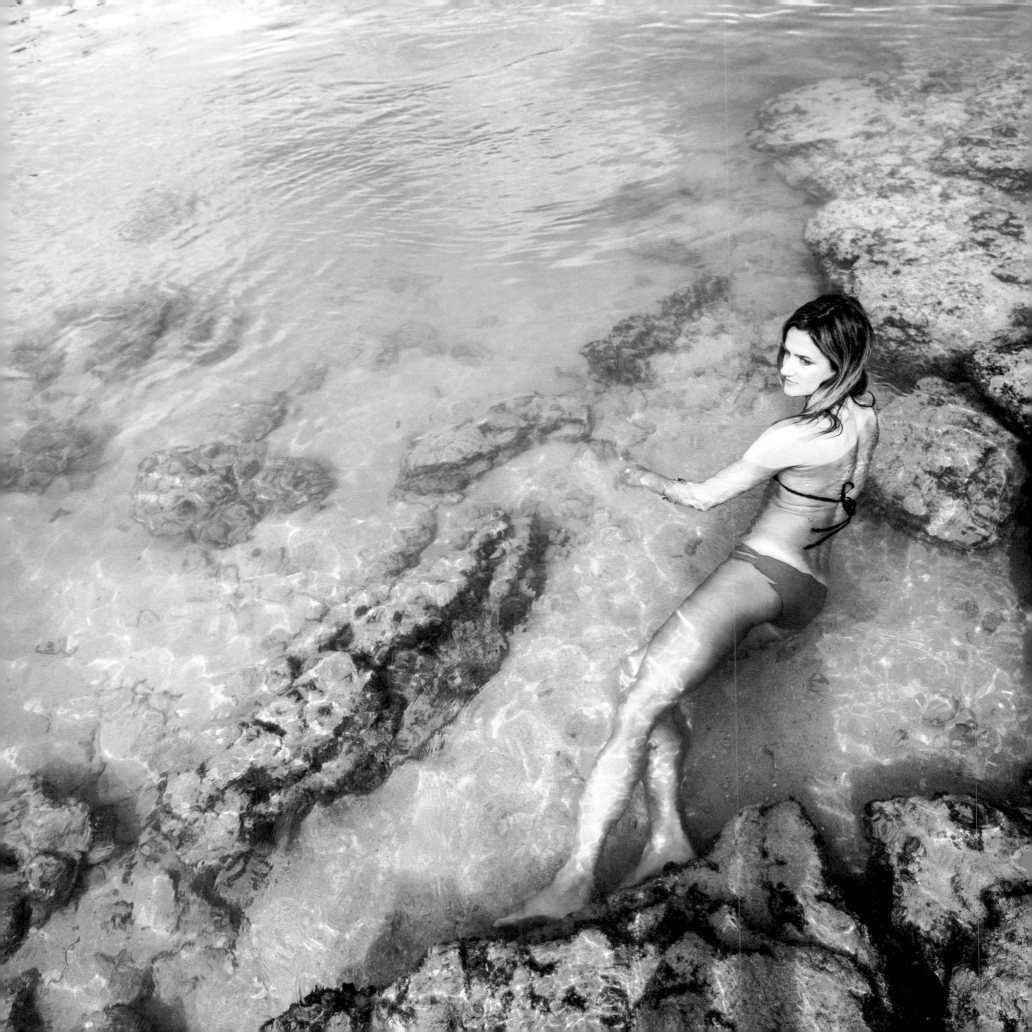

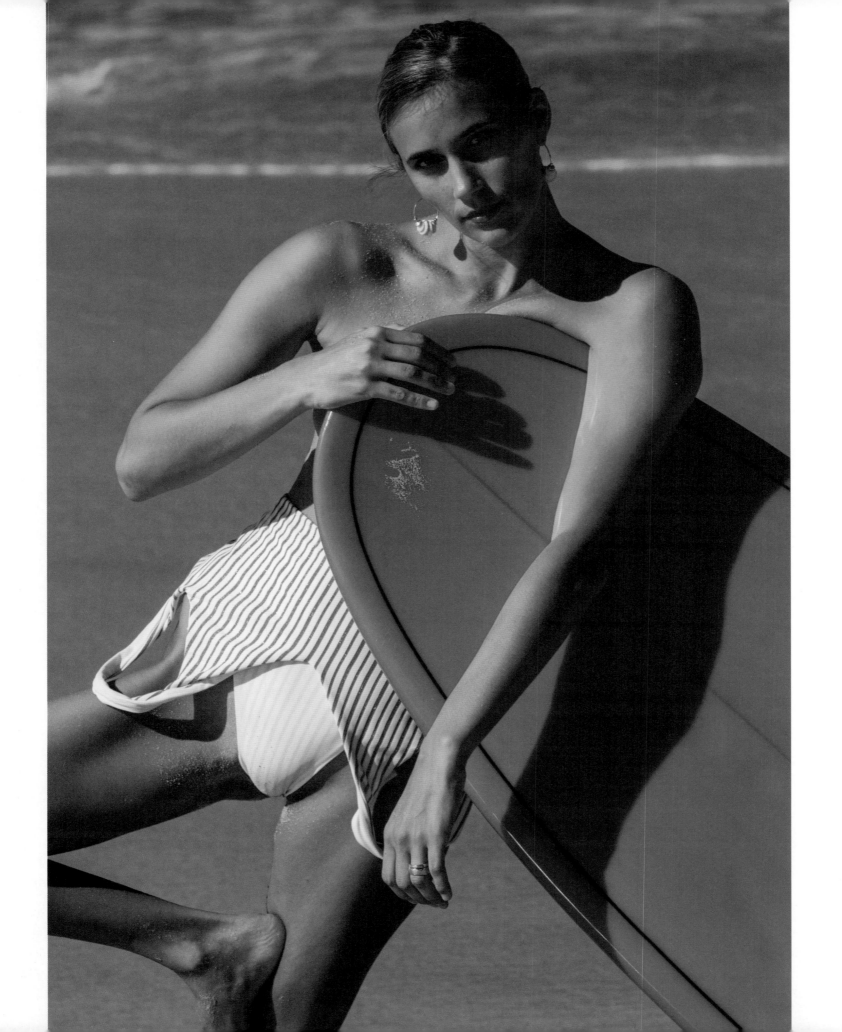

FOREWORD

Have you ever met someone that lights up the room when they walk through the door? That's Neely. I first met her at a mutual friend's house during a healthy living event. As soon as we began our conversation I thought to myself, I must know her secret. She radiates health and happiness, which inspired me to continue to pursue my goal of becoming my best possible self.

While I grew up training as a competitive athlete centered around physical health, when I became a physician and mother I started to branch out to learn about all aspects of wellness including nutritional and spiritual health. In addition, as I continued to treat patients every day, I realized that my Western medicine training was not structured to encompass all of these facets. I started to truly pay attention to the people who inspire me the most, and how they were radiating at a higher frequency than others. I suddenly understood how much knowledge and experience Neely had to offer, as well as the importance of her vision for this book. It seemed as though the power of the universe was shining upon us.

Project You links together all aspects of health, from nutrition to exercise, to mental health and meditation. As a physician, I believe the future of medicine will be in biogenomic identification, and this book uses evolutionary theory to make healthy choices applicable to your everyday life. Neely not only explains 'why' and gives the 'how', but also provides outstanding recipes that bring a whole new light to familiar ideas such as smoothies and soup bowls. You'll also find a comprehensive list of all things from superfoods to anti-aging skin and hair hacks, workout sessions, recipes, meditation guides and inspiring athlete's interpretations of health.

This book will serve as an ongoing resource for not only myself but my family and patients. It will be something to return to again and again, whether for a superfood-friendly recipe or for some tips on exercise and sleep. It really is a guide for all things "health", and relevant for whatever part of your journey to health that you are currently on.

April Mancuso Reynolds, DO
Board certified in Physical Medicine and Rehabilitation

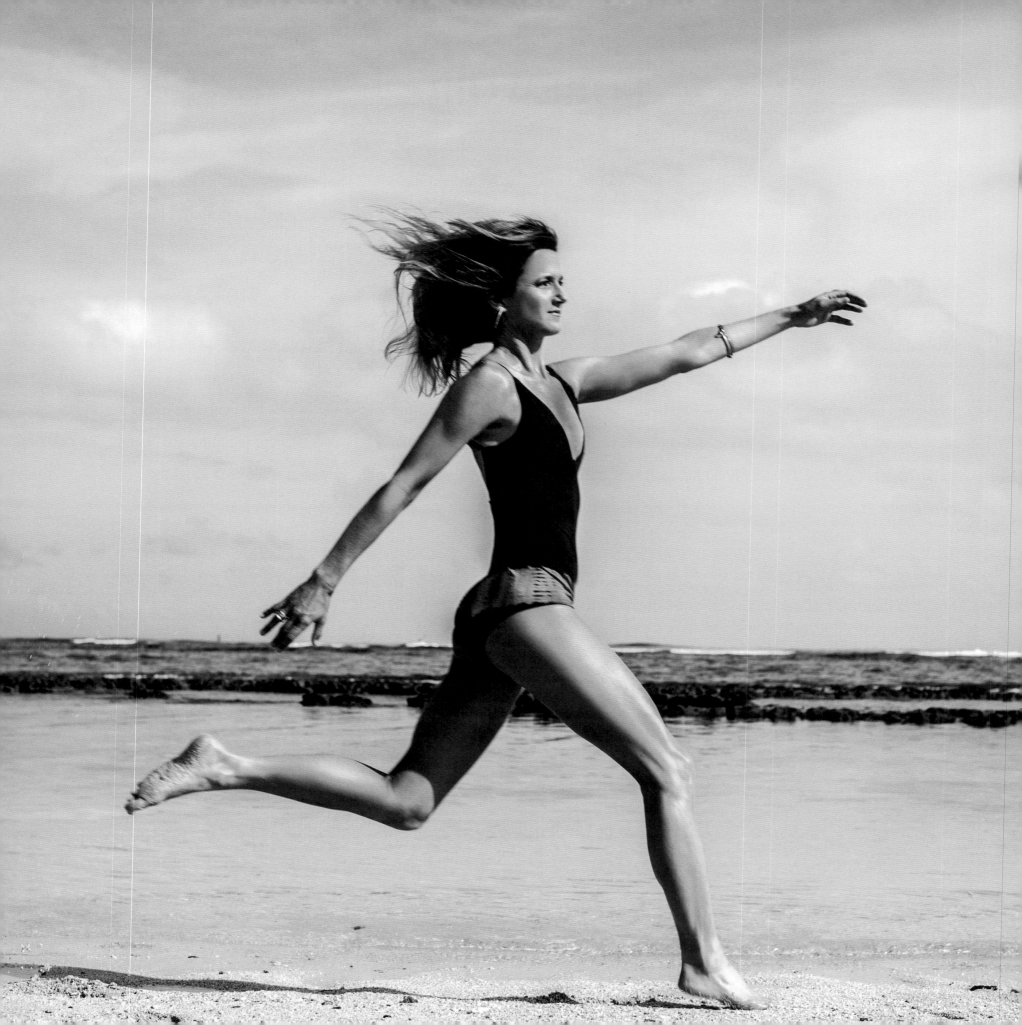

INTRODUCTION

My personal journey

I have been fascinated with health and longevity for as long as I can remember. I was a competitive tennis player from the age of eight, so working out, eating right and being at the top of my game was ingrained in my head at an early age. Also, I was afraid of dying. When I was 14 years old, I saw my cousin almost die from a severe drug and alcohol addiction, and I was determined to live a clean life. I had hope, as my great grandparents on my dad's side lived to 97 and 98, and my grandparents on the same side lived to 92 and 94.

I remained in excellent physical condition through my teen years and played competitive tennis in college. After college, my health began to deteriorate. My energy was consistently low and I was getting sick all the time. I didn't understand why. I was still exercising, playing sports and eating a healthy and balanced diet. Why was I feeling so horrible?

Thus began my lifelong quest to achieve what I call "true health," inside and out. When we discuss health in our society, it's usually in the context of physical health, which is why your annual doctor's appointment is referred to as a "physical." The questions that come up are things such as: Is your body disease-free? Injury-free? Are you exercising? Eating a well-balanced diet? Sleeping? You get the picture. Less consideration is given to the aspects of mental and spiritual health. But humans are more than just physical beings. We have a distinct mental and spiritual capacity that is interconnected with our bodies. Without attending to all of these components, we cannot achieve true health.

As my own health problems continued, I started to research societies where people lived long and healthy lives. I came upon an elite group of people who live to be over 110 years old, known as "supercentenarians." There are estimated 300 to 450 supercentenarians in the world, but only 47 verified cases are known.[1] They inhabit regions of the world defined by author Dan Buettner as "Blue Zones," [2] and include places such as Okinawa (Japan), Ikaria (Greece), Nicoya (Costa Rica), Sardinia (Italy) and Loma Linda (California). Buettner found that diet is the key to longevity in these areas – but he also found things such as sex, naps, wine, and time spent with good friends were key indicators of longevity. People in Blue Zones generally eat a plant-based diet, live in walkable communities, and live a life that is imbued with purpose. They are social and have a 'live in the present' mindset.

Living the kind of life that promotes longevity sounds well and good, but in today's fast-paced, "always on" world, it's easier said than done. After college, I found myself yearning to live a healthy and balanced life, but also scrambling to start a business, which left little time to work on my personal health and wellness. Despite the warnings and admonitions I received from friends and my family, at age 25 I dove head first into the cut-throat fashion world and launched my own leather accessories company. I didn't have the money or expertise to start a company, but I was determined to make it work and wouldn't listen to anyone who told me I couldn't. My business grew quickly, but so did my stress and anxiety. I suffered from insomnia for three months, which nearly crushed me. Around the same time, I met Philippe Colmant, a handsome young Microsoft engineer, who would become my business partner a year later, and my husband five years after that.

With Philippe at my side, my business stresses lessened, but my personal stresses grew. I tried for three years to get pregnant, which put tremendous stress on our marriage. I finally ended up getting pregnant at age 35 – with twins. We were thrilled and relieved, but I had no idea the physical and mental toll that raising two children would take on me. From there on out, it was almost impossible to find a healthy balance between motherhood, career and marriage. I tried to project the illusion of being a healthy, happy "super mom" while crushing it in the high fashion industry. But the truth was that I was struggling to get through each day. I was not sleeping enough, eating well, or taking care of myself. My anxiety level was sky high.

When I turned 40, by all appearances I was living the ideal life. I had two healthy kids, I was married to a great guy, and I was living the entrepreneurial dream as an accessories designer. But my quest for true health had been put on the back burner. I was struggling with several health issues, including extreme fatigue, hair loss and gastrointestinal issues. I backed off from work a little, slept more and spent more time cooking and gardening so that I could focus on healthy eating right from my garden. This should all equal more energy, right? No, instead I felt like a dead woman walking.

I vaguely remembered being anemic through college during my competitive tennis-playing years. My doctors told me I needed to eat more meat, which was a huge problem for me as I hated red meat. But I decided it was time to get my blood panels done. The results were alarming: my iron count was very low and my B12 was extremely low.

I made an appointment with a nutritionist, which worried me because the "old school" nutritionists I had seen in the past worked from the government standardized (FDA) food pyramid, which is still not correct in my mind. But this nutritionist, Willie Victor,[3] was different. She tested my blood for food allergies, and the results were incredible. Besides being allergic to dairy and gluten, I learned I was intolerant to other healthy foods, such as ginger, kale and wild salmon. Who would have guessed? We made modifications to my diet and eliminated all possible foods that might be causing inflammation.

This was a turning point for me. With Willie's help, I began to understand the amazing connection between our gut and intestinal health and our overall health. Who would have guessed that some of the very foods I thought were so healthy for me were tearing apart my gut, hurting my body and messing with my moods? I spent six weeks eliminating all of the inflammation-causing foods from my diet – all grains, sugar and dairy. As my gut healed, my energy returned to a level I hadn't felt since childhood, and my brain fog dissipated. I noticed I wasn't getting sick anymore. This all happened without the use of medication or the help of traditional Western doctors.

After I had my gut issues under control, I started working on my mental health. Juggling career, marriage and kids was taking a toll on me. The more I worked on being the "perfect" mom and having the "perfect" family, the more my work would suffer. When I refocused my energy on my work, my family would miss out. I realized I couldn't "have it all". I was anxious, depressed, and my marriage was crumbling.

I started taking trips by myself, where I tried to regain balance, strength and insight. I found that embracing nature – especially gliding and paddling through the beautiful blue waters as I surfed, gave me a sense of peace and hope. During my solo trips, I taught myself how to meditate and diligently practiced meditation twice every day. Through these moments of calm reflection, I became stronger and learned how to find balance within myself even when everything on the outside was going haywire.

My quest for true health is far from over. Each day, I work on the three pillars – internal (nutrition and gut health), physical (exercise and sleep) and emotional and spiritual self-care – that encourage my body to act and feel young. I invite you to join me in my journey.

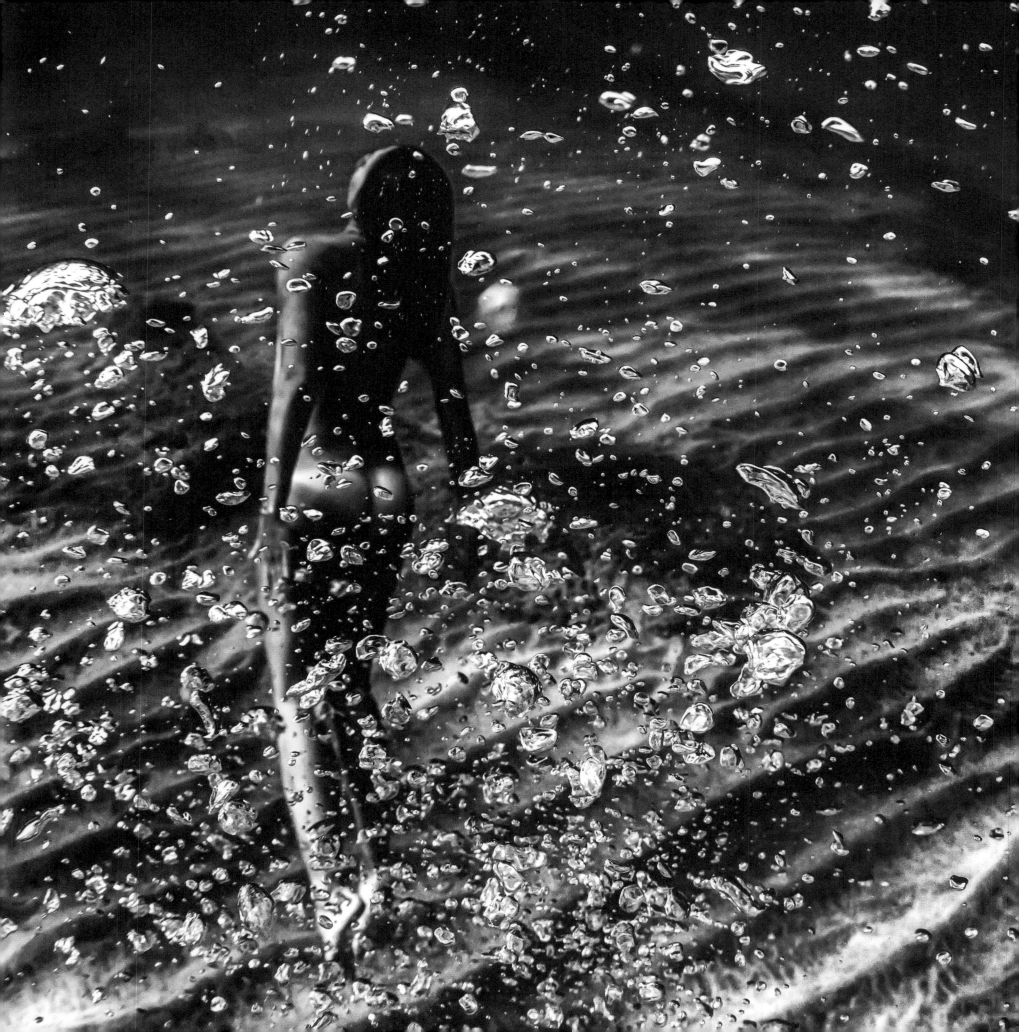

JOIN ME IN MY QUEST FOR TRUE HEALTH AND LONGEVITY

Project You is not another book about the latest fad diet or juice "cleanse". It is about living a clean and healthy life that will set you on the path to longevity. I am here to help you every step of the way through my amazing superfood recipes, exercise tips, and spiritual and mental wellness guidance. The fundamental purpose of this book is to show you how these pieces need to be connected in order for you to be 100 percent nourished inside and out. Come explore and live this intricate web of wellness in my book, *Project You.*

THE FOUR PRINCIPLES THIS BOOK WILL TEACH YOU

ONE: *The importance of superfoods & how to use them*

I will teach you how to make over 100 delicious, nutritionally dense superfood smoothies and soups right in your own kitchen. Learn what a superfood is and how to use it wisely for your body. I will list the nutritional value of over 25 super greens, 50 super fruits and 25 of the most powerful raw superfoods, nuts and seeds needed for a long healthy life – all of which I use in my smoothies and soups.

TWO: *The secrets to glowing skin & hair*

I share the key secrets and science to obtaining glowing skin and hair by combining nutritionally dense food with clean skin care products. I explain the importance of pure alkaline water and the amount of minerals needed each day for your body, and the connection water has to your health, gut, skin and hair. I also cover the importance of omega-3s, plant protein and how much you need for a mostly vegetarian diet.

THREE: *Exercise tips & simple workout routines*

I recommend a few weekly workout schedules and the necessary amount and type of exercise needed for your complete health, and why too much exercise could be lowering your immunity overall. I introduce a powerful photographic collection of female athletes and what wellness means to them.

FOUR: *Daily practices for mental & spiritual wellness*

What is the real story behind inner peace and longevity, and how do we achieve it? I share tips on how to achieve emotional balance through daily meditation practices, the power of touch and other healing, stress-relieving practices.

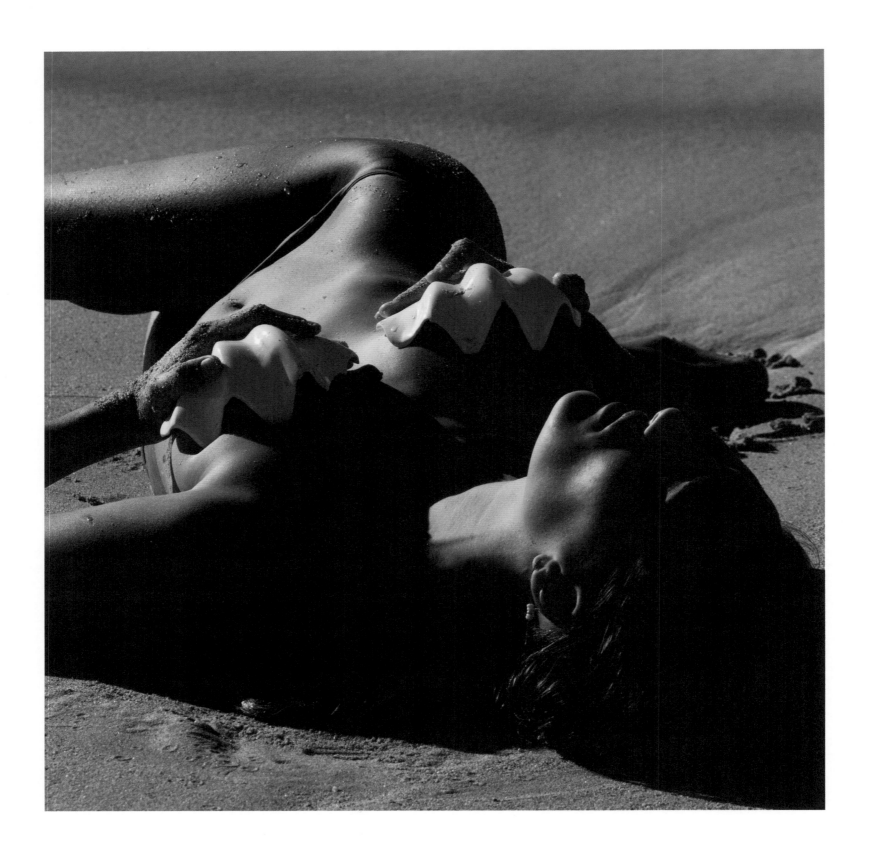

TABLE OF CONTENTS

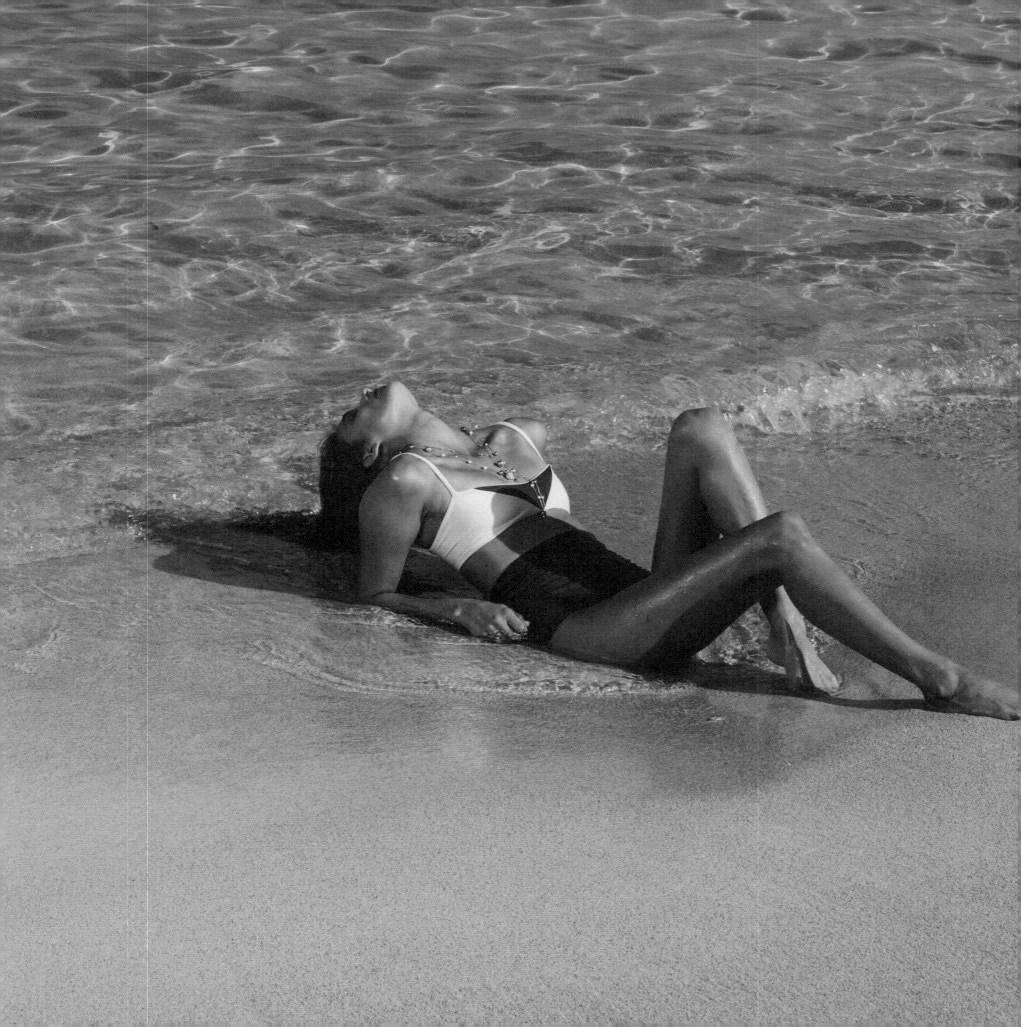

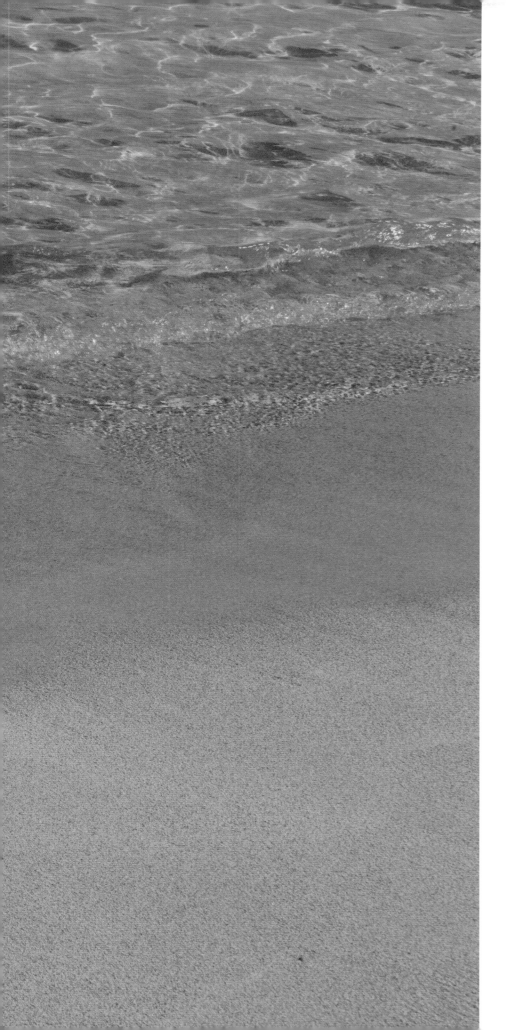

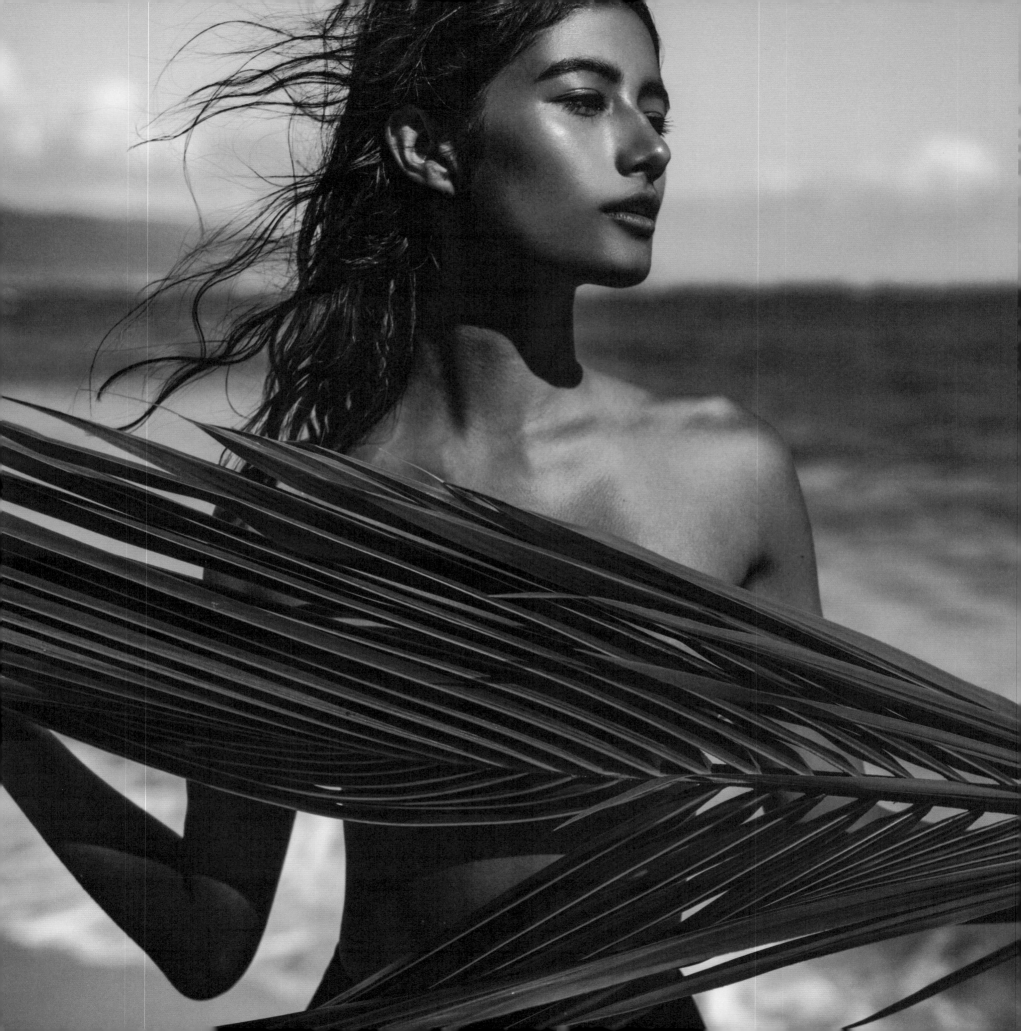

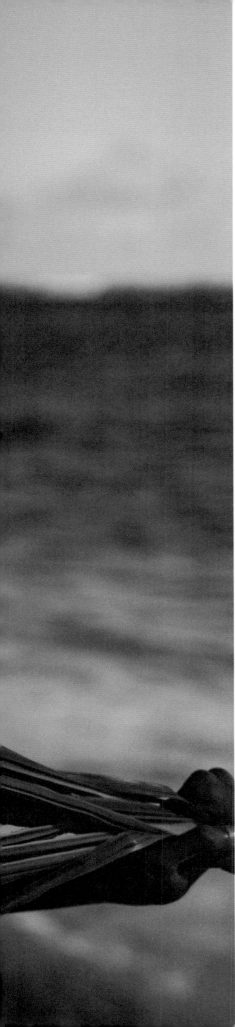

Chapter 1

MY GUT FEELING

You can dedicate your life to a healthy routine: you exercise, eat right, practice mindfulness and try to get enough sleep – but what if all that hard work was being sabotaged by poor gut health?

I decided to separate out the discussion of gut health – the role our digestive system plays in our overall well-being – from the nutrition section of the book because it is an important topic that I believe deserves its own category. I discovered I was suffering from what is called "leaky gut syndrome" this past year, when I visited Willie Victor – a nutritional consultant in Mill Valley, California, who specializes in helping clients suffering from autoimmune and inflammatory diseases. She explained to me that leaky gut is a condition where the intact walls of the intestines develop tiny holes, allowing penetration of bacteria, toxins and food into the bloodstream that can lead to serious health problems. It can also cause what is called "brain fog," a commonly used phrase to describe feelings of confusion, forgetfulness, and lack of focus and mental clarity.

It was hard for me to believe I was suffering from leaky gut since my diet was so incredibly clean, consisting mainly of wholegrains, fruit and vegetables and protein. But I had been experiencing severe inflammation in both of my knees, to the point where I could not exercise or even walk without pain. I had already had one operation for a meniscus tear a few years before.

Willie explained to me that my knee pain might be caused by my intestinal issues. Recent research has shown the connection between digestive problems and diseases such as rheumatoid arthritis (RA).[4] She did a blood test that checked for food allergies, and the results were fascinating. They showed I was allergic to dairy and gluten, which wasn't a huge surprise since these are common food allergies for many people. More surprisingly, the tests revealed I was intolerant to foods that I thought were healthy, such as ginger, kale and wild salmon. We made modifications to my diet and eliminated all possible foods that might be causing inflammation.

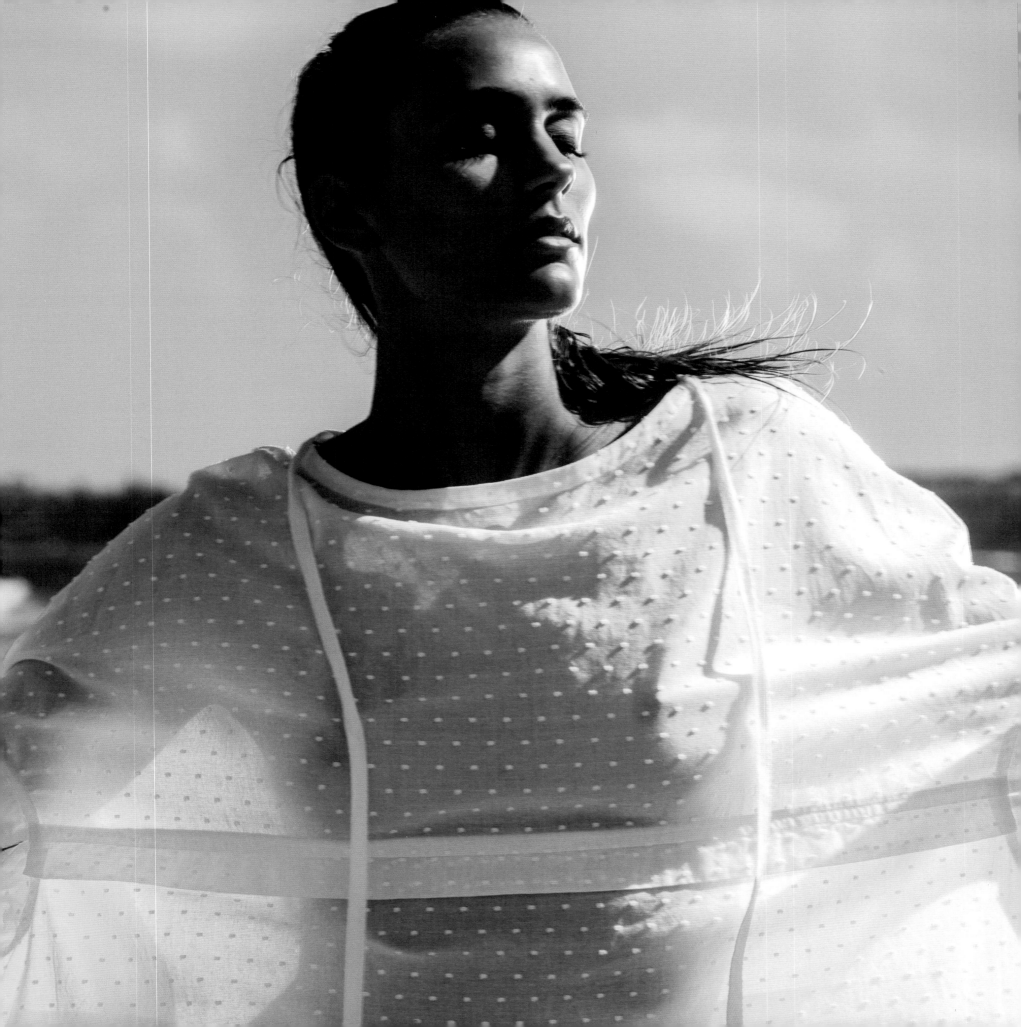

Chapter 2

WHAT IS GUT HEALTH, ANYWAY?

While it has been known for ages that food can be either the best medicine or a strong poison to your body, what hasn't been understood well until recently is the role that gut health plays in our overall wellbeing – physical, mental and emotional. You can think of your gut as your body's second brain.[5] If your gut health is poor, you can end up with impaired immune and nervous systems, autoimmune diseases and distressed hormonal function throughout the body. This is because our gastrointestinal tract is loaded with neurons that release the same neurotransmitters found in the brain. Any upset to this equilibrium can throw your body and mood into chaos.

As your skin forms a barrier to the outside world, your gut plays a similar role inside your body. Your gut acts as a gatekeeper that filters out the toxic substances that enter your digestive tract, and allows in the nutrients that build your muscles and tissues. The gut is in continuous contact with nutrients, as well as toxins, food additives, microbes and pharmaceuticals that might pass through your digestive tract on a daily basis.

Inside a healthy gut lives a world of friendly bacteria that help us digest food, produce vitamins and short-chain fats, stimulate a vibrant gut lining and keep unfriendly organisms in check. According to Dr. Vincent Pedre in his book, *Happy Gut* [6], a healthy gut is one where:

- All food is digested into its component parts.
- The digestive surface is vibrant and able to absorb all of the important micronutrients your body needs while blocking the entrance of larger, partially un-digested food particles, bacteria, yeast, parasites, antibiotics and pesticides.
- The gut-associated immune system is activated only when necessary and is not over-stimulated.

You have to know what is in the foods you eat if you want to have a healthy gut. For example, if you are having stomach problems, it may be due to the processed foods or foods your body sees as foreign "toxins" that cause inflammation in your body. According to Dr. Pedre, what you eat can actually turn on or off good and bad genes.[7] For example, eating steamed broccoli can "turn on" anti-cancer and anti-inflammatory gene pathways, whereas processed foods that cause inflammation can "turn on" certain carcinogenic gene pathways.

AN UNHEALTHY GUT CAN LEAD TO AUTOIMMUNE DISEASES

While it's not commonly discussed in medical circles, research has shown that leaky gut syndrome is also linked to autoimmune problems.[8] Gut issues whether they're caused by food, stress or medication can result in inflammation that triggers the immune system, causing it to work overtime and become weakened. In response, certain triggers – which can be as small as a cold or as big as a birth, death or accident – can cause the body to self-attack. This can manifest in multiple ways throughout the body, including problems with the thyroid, bowels and joints.

STRESS: AN UNLIKELY CAUSE OF GUT DISTRESS

Stress is another common reason why your gut can be unhappy. Research shows the stress response in your body can literally change the natural balance of healthy bacteria in your gut, causing the gut ecology to change in favor of a more hostile group of bacteria.[9] I have learned the hard way, but now I make time every day to incorporate some type of stress management routine into my daily life, whether it's meditation, yoga or outdoor exercise.

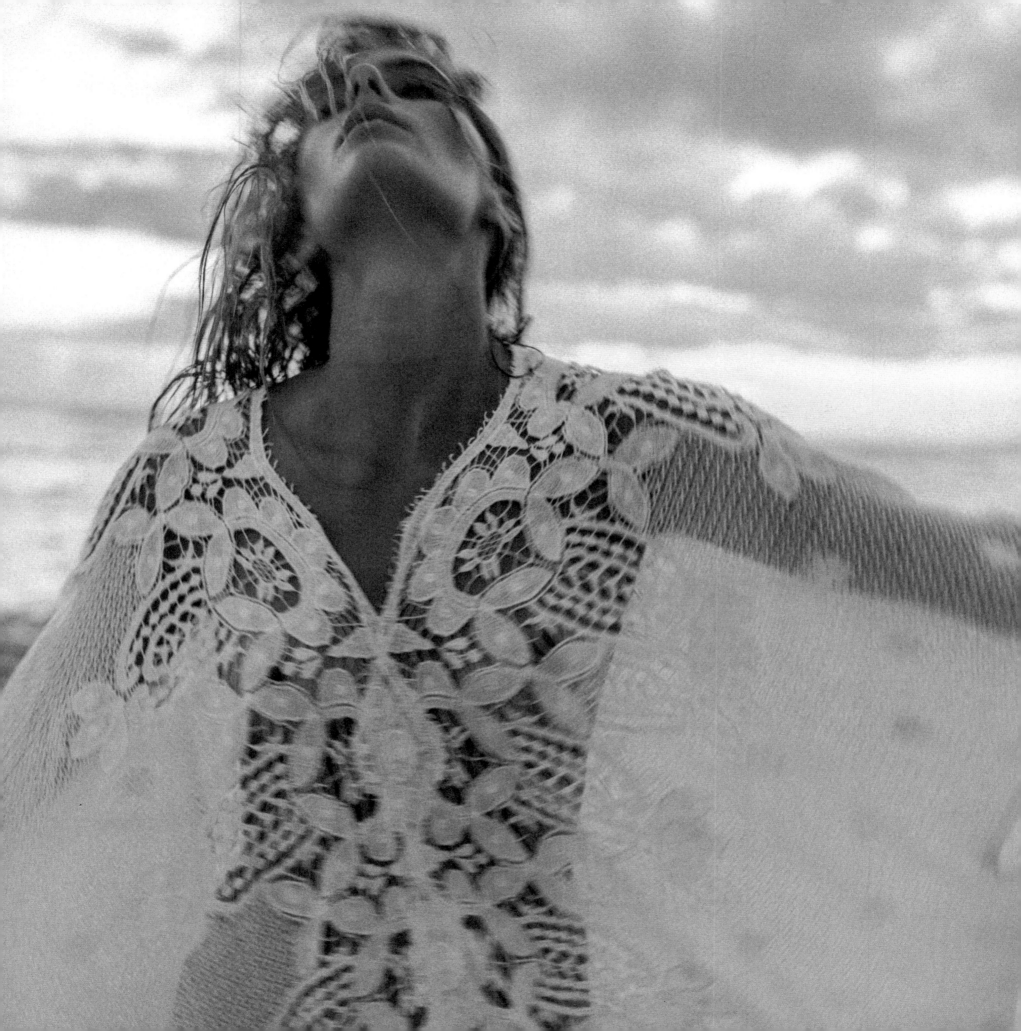

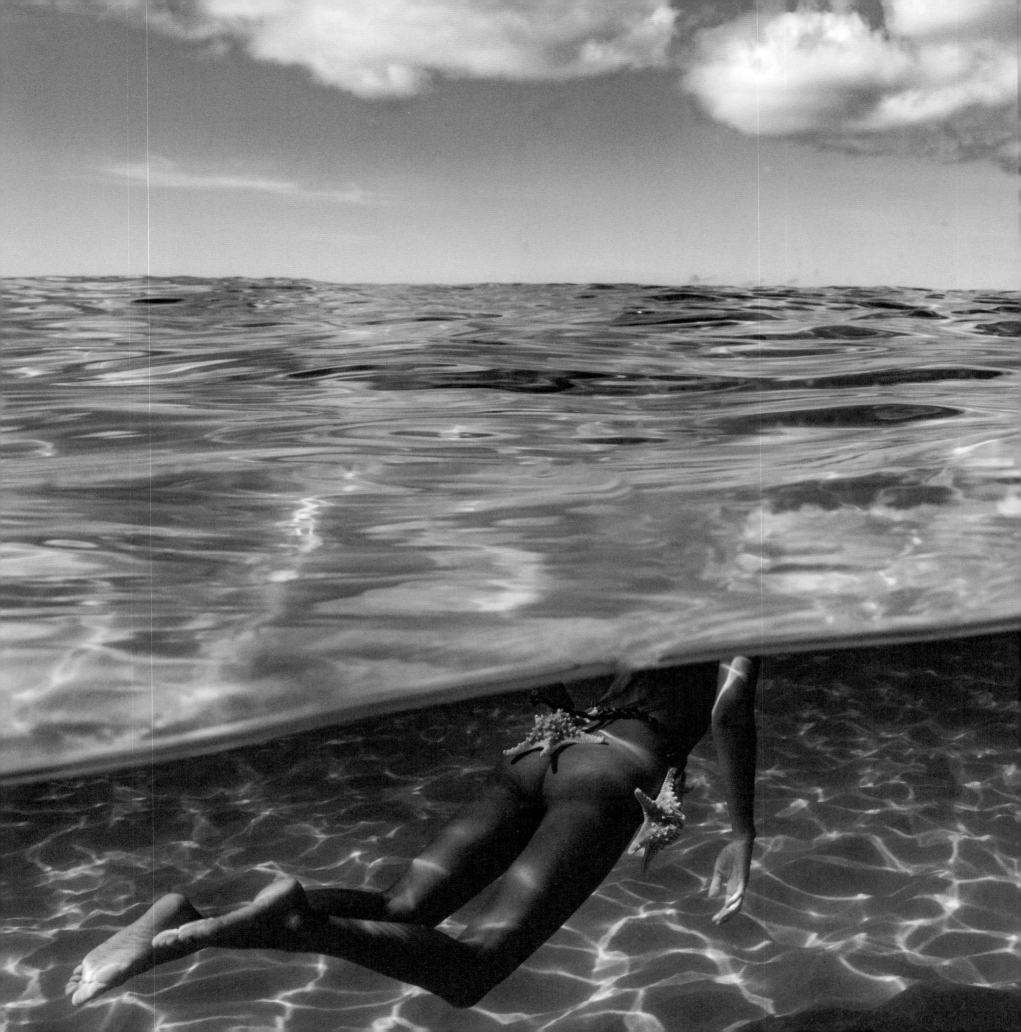

Chapter 3

HEALING A LEAKY GUT

To heal my leaky gut, I had to make changes to my diet, learn to manage my stress level, and get more sleep. Here, I share with you the clear and simple guidelines I used to heal my gut.[10]

STEP ONE: FIGURE OUT WHAT IS CAUSING YOUR LEAKY GUT

Possible Causes of Leaky Gut Syndrome

- **Food sensitivities** may require a blood test to be determined. Some common allergens include gluten, dairy and soy. Once you discover which foods are causing problems, you need to eliminate them from your diet to heal your gut.
- **Stress** causes the body to produce a lot of cortisol, which thins the lining of the gut. The thinner the lining of the gut, the more the opportunity to have the gut leak. This can affect your villi (small finger-like projections of tissue contained in the small intestine that increase its surface area and aid in the absorption of particular nutrients).
- **Small intestine bacterial overgrowth (SIBO)** is where the colon bacteria seeps up into the small intestine where they should not be. It also releases a toxin that not only damages the gut, but slows down motor complexes, which can cause constipation, bloating and gassiness. SIBO is fed by particular foods, meaning it can grow if you are eating these foods. SIBO also starts to digest and consume a lot of important nutrients such as iron and B12, which then can become depleted, causing overall deficiencies and continued leaky gut syndrome.
- **Other parasites** or imbalances in gut flora can cause leaky gut syndrome.
- **Gluten** can also damage the villi (finger-like projections in the small intestine that help absorb our food more efficiently in the body) especially if you have celiac disease.
- **Medications and over-the-counter drugs**, including non-steroidal anti-inflammatory drugs (NSAIDs) such as Advil and Motrin (ibuprofen) and Aleve (naproxen), can compromise the gut lining and cause inflammation, the very problem that these drugs have been designed to help.

STEP TWO: REMOVE THE TRIGGER

- **Eliminate foods** causing allergies or sensitivities.
- **Work on stress management,** as daily stress adds up to high overall stress that will start to affect the gut. Use stress release methods such as meditation, massage or going for a walk.
- **Test for SIBO or other parasites**, especially traveler's diarrhea or food poisoning. Ask your doctor to test for IBS (Irritable Bowel Syndrome), especially if you have been traveling outside the US. This test will check for inflammation and determine if there is still some kind of bug left in your intestines. This test is typically done by a gastroenterologist.
- **Reduce the use of medications and over the counter drugs** such as ibuprofen and naproxen.

STEP THREE: ADD GUT-SUPPORTING SUPPLEMENTS TO YOUR DIET

- **Muciliginous herbs,** such as marshmallow root, slippery elm and comfrey with fenugreek, produce gel in the gut, which aids in its smoothing and healing.
- **Aloe** coats the gut and aids in the healing process. Use a form of aloe made from the inner leaf of the plant.
- **Turmeric and black pepper extract** help the entire body and gut tremendously by decreasing inflammation. Use turmeric under guidance of a practitioner, as there can be interactions with other medications.
- **Zinc** is a very important nutrient that helps tighten the villi and heal leaky gut.
- **L-glutamine** is an amino acid that is the primary fuel used by the cells in your gut lining for repair and regrowth.
- **Short-chain fatty acids (SCFA)** are important for building the lining of our gut but are excreted with good bacteria (in your stool). In some cases you will need to take supplements that will help build the wall of the gut by supplying SCFA.

STEP FOUR: TAKE THESE POINTS INTO CONSIDERATION

- **Eat small, regular meals** and do not let long periods of time go by without food.
- **Alkalize your diet** by eating at least seven servings of dark vegetable greens a day along with three servings of fruit.
- **Chew food well**.
- **Support the gut with digestive enzymes** that aid in the breakdown of protein.

CHECK YOUR POOP!

Your poop is critical to how your body is working. What you eat and how you poop it out is how we eliminate toxins and repair and heal our body. You'll know your gut is working well if you have at least one bowel movement a day without strain. Your stool should be formed (not liquidy), smooth and easy to pass, and six inches or longer. Sounds disgusting, but this is incredibly important for our overall health.

ELIMINATION DIET*

The most common types of elimination diets involve removing specific foods or ingredients from your daily diet because they may be causing allergy symptoms. The basic elimination diet is as simple as this: Exclude all gluten, dairy, eggs, nuts, soy, sugar, fast food, and alcohol for about one month. So what are you supposed to eat? Eat 30 percent "clean" protein, such as organic, hormone-free, grass-fed lean beef, poultry and some wild clean fish.[12] 70 percent of your diet should be vegetables, legumes (e.g. beans and lentils), seeds, Arctic and Northern Atlantic seaweeds and gluten-free pseudograins such as quinoa.

After one month, you may reintroduce one irritant, such as gluten or dairy and see how you feel. If there is no reaction after two days, eat the same food again and notice how you feel for a second time. If all is good and you are having no negative reactions or side effects, you can keep eating this food. After this process, you may pick another food to reintroduce. Follow the same process with each food that has been eliminated. If you are working with a nutritionist or doctor, you can take a blood test that will reveal which foods you have most sensitivity to. These immediate foods will need to be excluded along with the list above. The reintroduction process is the same process as the above.[13]

*We advise that any type of elimination diet is done while under the supervision of a medical professional or nutritionist.

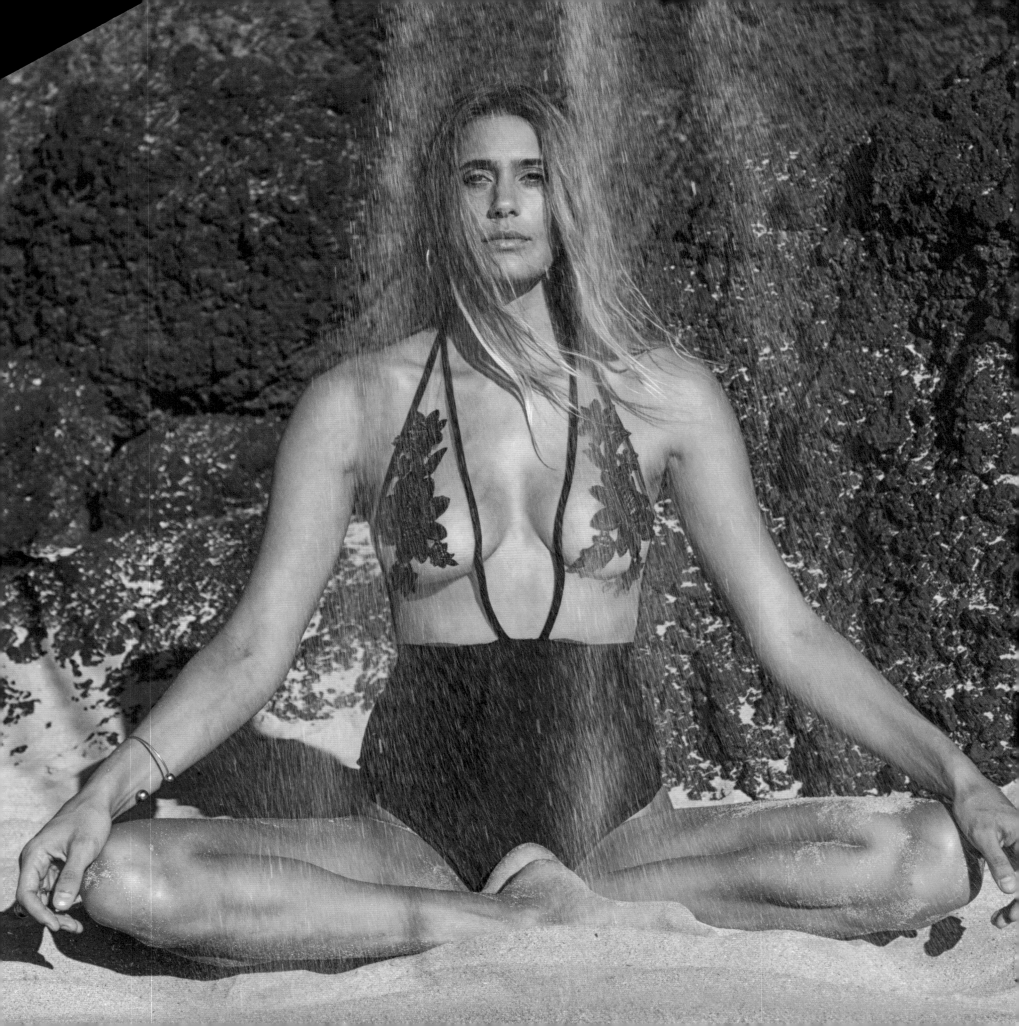

BRAIN FOG

Cognitive dysfunction, otherwise known as brain fog, is characterized by feelings of confusion, forgetfulness, a lack of focus and mental clarity, and poor concentration. Almost everyone has experienced or suffered from it at some point in their life, and although it's common, it is not normal or healthy.

Brain fog can be caused by lifestyle factors such as diet, stress, or lack of sleep or exercise. In other situations, it can be indicative of a serious underlying health condition. It's important to be aggressive about adopting a brain-healthy lifestyle and managing your daily nutritional habits. Adding our superfood smoothies and soups to your everyday diet is a great way to jump-start your body in the right direction.[11]

There are innumerable causes of brain fog. Finding your personal brain fog solution will take time and some trial and error. Here is a checklist to get started.

- **A food elimination diet** or food sensitivity test is the best place to start.
- **Include healthy fats** in your diet. Nuts, Ahiflower oil, olive oil, coconut oil, avocado and sardines are all nutritional necessities for a healthy brain.
- **Drink enough water** – try to average eight 12-ounce bottles of clean spring water a day.
- **Get adequate sleep** – eight hours is a perfect amount to shoot for.
- **Exercise** is important as it increases the blood flow, oxygen and nutrients your brain needs and this can sharpen up your brain quickly.
- **Meditate** as this reduces stress and clears the mind allowing you to become clear and calm.
- **Talk to your doctor about changing prescriptions** or over the counter medications or minimizing your dosage. Statins (cholesterol-lowering drugs) and sleeping pills are examples of medications that cause brain fog memory loss.
- **Eliminate toxins from your home and surrounding environment**, as we all currently live in a sea of untested chemicals that get absorbed directly into our body. Molds, dust, pet dander, polychlorinated biphenyls (or PCBs, a family of highly toxic chemical compounds), home cleaning products and off-gassing from mattresses and carpets are just a few of many ways that toxins get caught in our homes. This pool of chemicals can cause major brain fog. I recommend switching to a natural mattress, purchasing carpets or rugs that are 100 percent wool or cotton, or getting rid of carpets all together. All toxic house cleaners should be thrown out immediately. I suggest only using plain vinegar and biodegradable soap and lemon to clean your entire house. Test your house for mold and keep dust to a bare minimum.

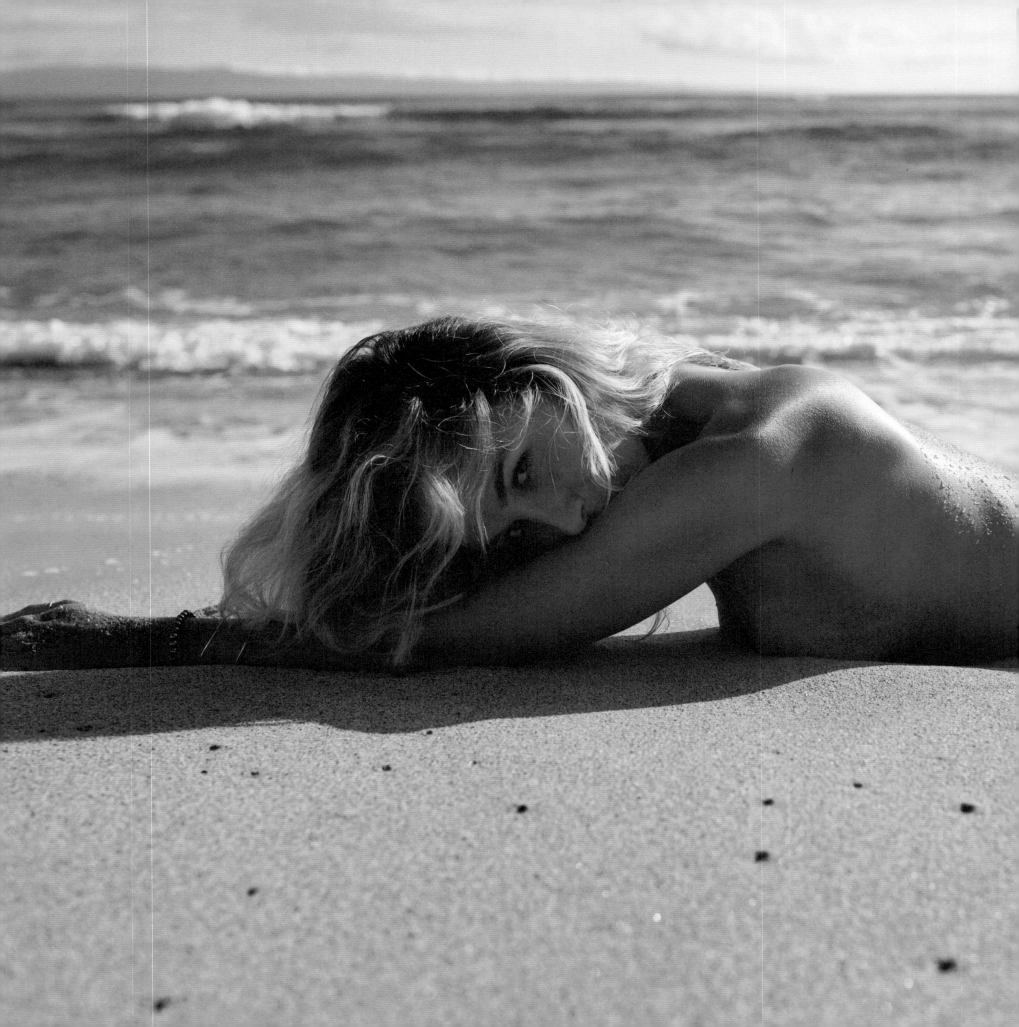

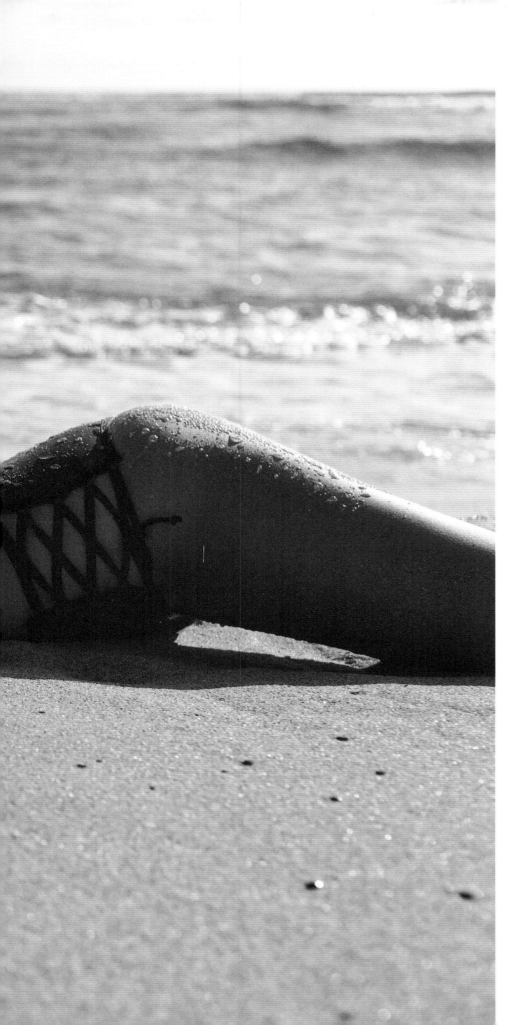

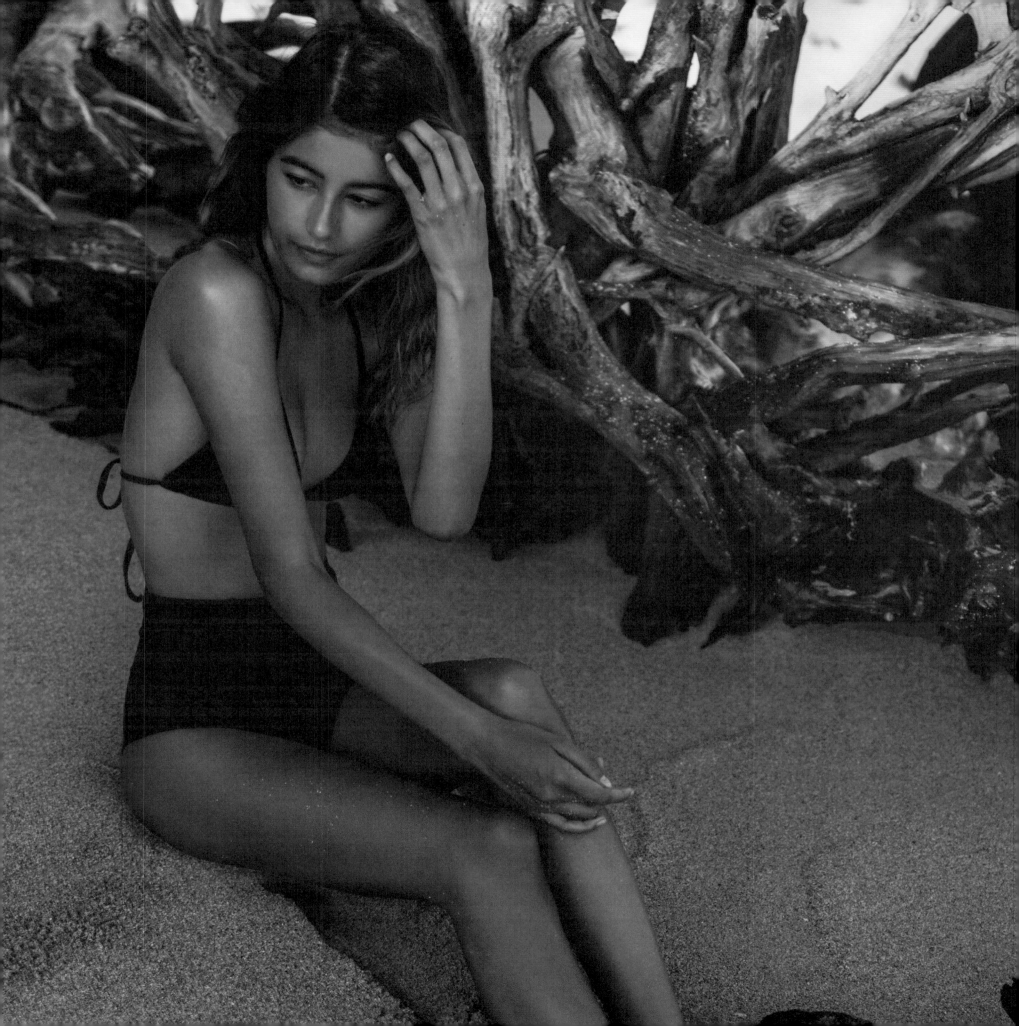

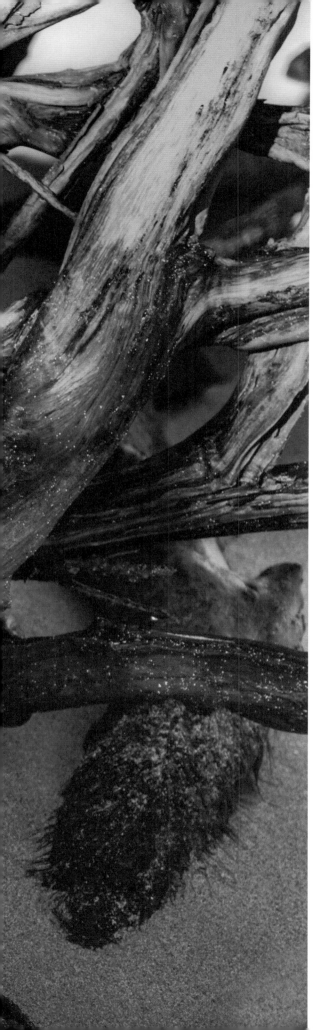

Chapter 4

WHY SUPERFOODS?

Superfoods are foods packed with very highly concentrated amounts of vitamins, minerals and antioxidants. Most superfoods pack a big punch, meaning you only have to eat a handful to get an enormous amount of nutrients, including essential vitamins such as A, B, C, D, E and K, and minerals such as calcium, iron, potassium, magnesium, zinc and enzymes.

How do superfoods promote true health and longevity? First, these foods are naturally rich in antioxidants, which help fight off free radicals in our body. Free radicals are unstable molecules that react quickly with essential molecules in our body (such as DNA, fat and proteins) causing cell damage. Free radical damage is linked with diseases such as cancer and heart disease, accelerated aging and a host of autoimmune diseases.[14] Free radicals are formed as part of our natural metabolism but can also be caused by environmental factors such as smoking, pesticides, pollution and radiation. Foods that are very high in antioxidants have been shown to neutralize or cancel out free radical damage to our cells and body over all.[15]

The easiest way to incorporate superfoods into your diet is to blend them into the antioxidant-rich smoothies and soups I outline in chapters seven to nine in this book. These smoothies also include important fibers that can help lower your cholesterol, keep your blood sugar stable, make it easier to lose weight, and even keep you alive longer. Since fiber cannot be broken down and absorbed by your digestive system, it moves through your body, slowing down and making your stools softer and easier to pass.

There are two types of fiber that your body needs: soluble and insoluble. Both come from plants and are forms of carbohydrates. Foods that include **soluble fibers** gel up in water, such as seeds, psyllium husk from the seed, chia from the seed, hemp seed, flax seed and apple pectin through apples. These fibers have different, yet equally important, nutritional components than super leafy greens. Your body also needs **insoluble fiber** from foods such as oats, legumes (peas, beans, lentils), and fruits such as oranges and apples that do not absorb or dissolve in water. Insoluble fiber is lost when you juice fruits and vegetables, which strains out important nutrients needed to detoxify the body.

Some of the very **powerful superfoods** I use in my nutritionally dense smoothies and soups include Australian superfoods, such as kakadu plum powder (a fruit with the highest form of vitamin C in the world), davidson plum powder, quandong powder, riberry powder, raw cacao powder, raw cacao nibs, camu powder, moringa, maca root powder, chlorella, spirulina, E3Live blue-green algae, sacha inchi powder, maqui powder, raw hemp seeds, raw sesame seeds, wheatgrass powder, goji berries and noni powder.

Some of the **super greens** I like to work with are raw spinach, romaine lettuce, kale, arugula, super greens mix, butter and red lettuces, cilantro, Italian flat parsley, celery, fresh mint and spearmint, bok choy, Swiss chard and artichoke. For my golden smoothies I like working with pumpkin (all types), yams, sweet potatoes and acorn squash, since they are packed with carotenoids and antioxidants.

Everyday fruits I like to use in my smoothies are kiwi, pear, lemon, dates, banana, apple, mango, plums, pluots (fruits that are 70 percent plum and 30 percent apricots), strawberries, blueberries, peaches, persimmons, pineapple, tangerine, raspberries, satsuma orange, cherries, rhubarb, goji berries, watermelon, cantaloupe and papaya. I also like to step outside the box and have fun using some powerful fruits from around the world such as green sapote, cactus pear, guava and dragon fruit.

EATING FROM YOUR GARDEN

It is important to know where your food is coming from. I want people to understand that eating is really a way of life. It's not dieting, but rather learning how to live a long and healthy life. My grandmother, Elaine, had the most amazing gardens filled with superfoods that she used to cook her meals. It's no surprise that both she and my grandfather lived into their mid-90s. Growing your own food or at least knowing where your food comes from is a big step in the right direction in attaining true health. Anyone can garden, no matter where they live. Gardening forces you to slow down and live in the present, two other components that lead to longevity. You can grow plants in pots outside on your deck or on your rooftop if you live in a city. If you don't want to tend your own garden, you can shop at your local farmers market or order farm boxes that can be delivered from local organic farms right to your front door.

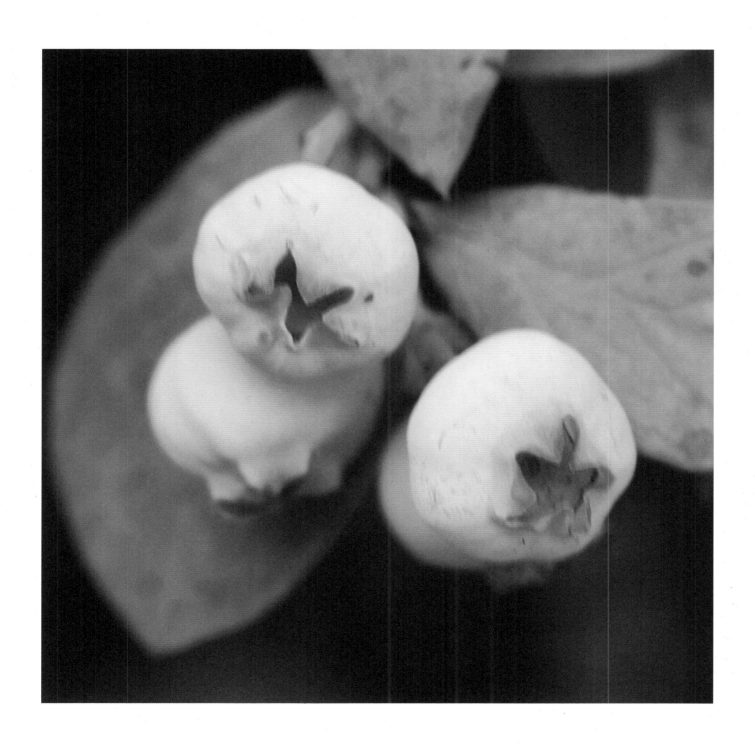

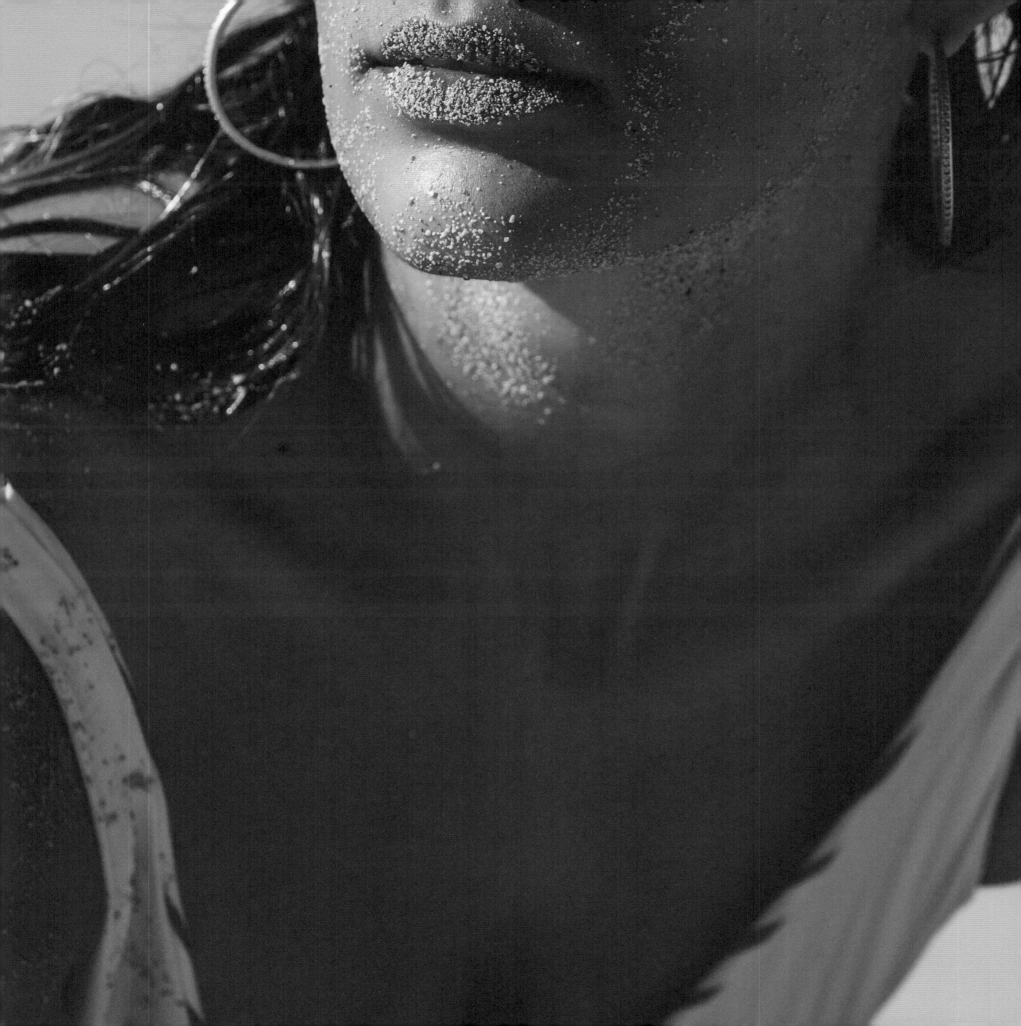

Chapter 5

AUSTRALIAN "FAB FOUR" SUPERFOODS

I searched the globe for sustainable superfoods, many of which have been forgotten or are even undiscovered. When I was living in Australia, I became familiar with the Indigenous Australian culture, which includes some of the oldest living people on Earth. The Aboriginal people have lived off their land for over 50,000 years, finding joy and sustenance from eating their own native superfoods grown right in their backyard. Because they use only what they need to survive, there is still an abundance of these vitamin-packed Aussie superfoods available.

The very ancient family of Australian superfoods are not known to most of the world. I will describe them and tell you where you can find them so you can include them in the smoothies and soups you make at home.

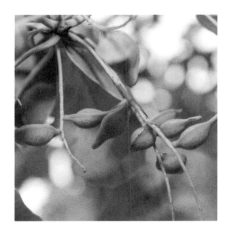

KAKADU PLUM

The kakadu plum is Australia's most potent superstar of superfoods. This pale pear-green colored oval fruit has a wooden, stone-like kernel, with a fibrous texture and tart and bitter flavor. It is packed with vitamin C and has some of the strongest medicinal properties of any food source. It has 100 times more vitamin C than an orange and five times higher antioxidant capability than a blueberry.[16]

Its medicinal uses are endless. The fruit has been used as an antiseptic and healing remedy by the indigenous people for thousands of years. After harvesting season the tree sap has been used to treat joint inflammation, while the tree bark is applied to the body and may help treat burns, rashes and infections. The kakadu plum contains phytochemicals such as gallic and ellagic acids. Gallic acid has been found to have antibacterial, antiviral and antifungal properties and also shows anti-inflammatory, antitumor, antimutagenic and anti-bronchodilatory activities. Ellagic acid has anti-carcinogenic effects against a wide range of carcinogens in many human tissues.[17]

While there are other fruits that contain antioxidants, the kakadu plum is unique because it contains both hydrophilic (water-soluble) and lipophilic (oil-soluble) antioxidants. This combination of antioxidants is much more bioavailable to the skin and body, delivering more comprehensive protection from oxidative stress than fruits comprised of only hydrophilic compounds. Kakadu plum also contains folate (vitamin B9), which plays a key role in repair and synthesis of DNA and can help to protect cells from damage. With its rich composition of phytochemicals and microelements, the kakadu plum is a powerful weapon that can help prevent premature aging.

The kakadu plum has many other names depending on where it's grown, such as gubinge, gabiny, kabiny, mardorr plum or murunga, bush plum, billygoat and salty plum. I use this fruit in almost all of my smoothies and some of my soups in the form of kakadu plum powder product, which is derived from certified organic, wild-harvested fruit. (See the *Resources* section for where to buy the powder).

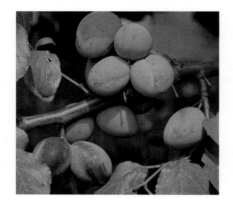

DAVIDSON PLUM

The davidson plum is a dark blue or purple-colored super fruit on the outside with a deep blood-reddish color on the inside. It contains high levels of anthocyanins, antioxidants that combat cell damage and help to prevent or delay Alzheimer's, heart disease, stroke, cancer, diabetes and gum disease. Its antioxidant capacity is much higher than a blueberry, which means we can eat smaller amounts and still receive all of the nutritional benefits. Because of their bitter taste, these plums are often not eaten as a fresh fruit, but they are great fruit for making jams and jellies. They have strong fruit acids and low sugar content, which provide additional health benefits. This plum was widely used by the indigenous culture. Following European settlement, they were eaten fresh and sometimes dipped in salt and sugar to achieve that sweet and sour combo.

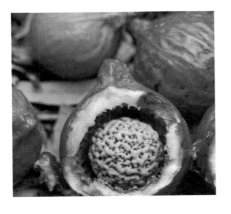

QUANDONG

Quandong, also known as the desert peach or wild peach, is a small native Australian shrub that grows seven to twenty feet. Quandongs are glossy, crimson fruits with a tart, slightly sweet and tangy taste. Quandong was a significant source of protein, vitamin C, E, folate, magnesium, calcium, iron, rutin and zinc for the indigenous Pitjantjatjara people, an Indigenous Australian clan of the Central Australian desert, for over 50,000 years and is still eaten by many of the people today. It's a rich source of phenolic-based antioxidants, which boost the immune system and protect against a number of illnesses such as cardiovascular disease, cancer and Alzheimer's. The fruits are made up of 25 percent protein and 70 percent complex oils and the kernels of the fruit were used by local clans to create powerful antibacterial and anti-inflammatory pastes. Because of its high content of protein, the Pitjantjatjara men would consider this a great substitute for meat. The leaves and bark from the trees would then be used mostly for medicinal purposes. Today quandong is also used for treating skin conditions and rheumatism. I include a delicious Quandong Peach Smoothie in the *Smoothie* section.

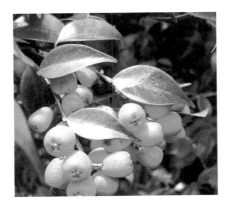

RIBERRY

Riberry, aka the lilly pilly, is a pear-shaped fruit a little over half an inch in length. It bares a bright cherry-red color that fades to pink when cooked and is native to the sub-tropical areas in Queensland and New South Wales. For thousands of years, Indigenous Australians on the east coast relied on the riberry as a core food source.

Riberry has three times the folate (B12) as blueberries, and is rich in manganese, and an important vegan source of calcium. Like the davidson plum, riberries contain high amounts of anthocyanins that combat cell damage, improve cognitive function, protect against cancers, heart and Alzheimer's diseases. Riberries provide an abundance of essential vitamins and minerals to fight against common colds and help to keep the immune system strong and healthy. These fruits were originally harvested by Aboriginal women and children. While children thought of the berries as sweet treats, adults referred to them as "medicine berries". They have a refreshingly tart and spicy flavor with a hint of cloves or cinnamon.

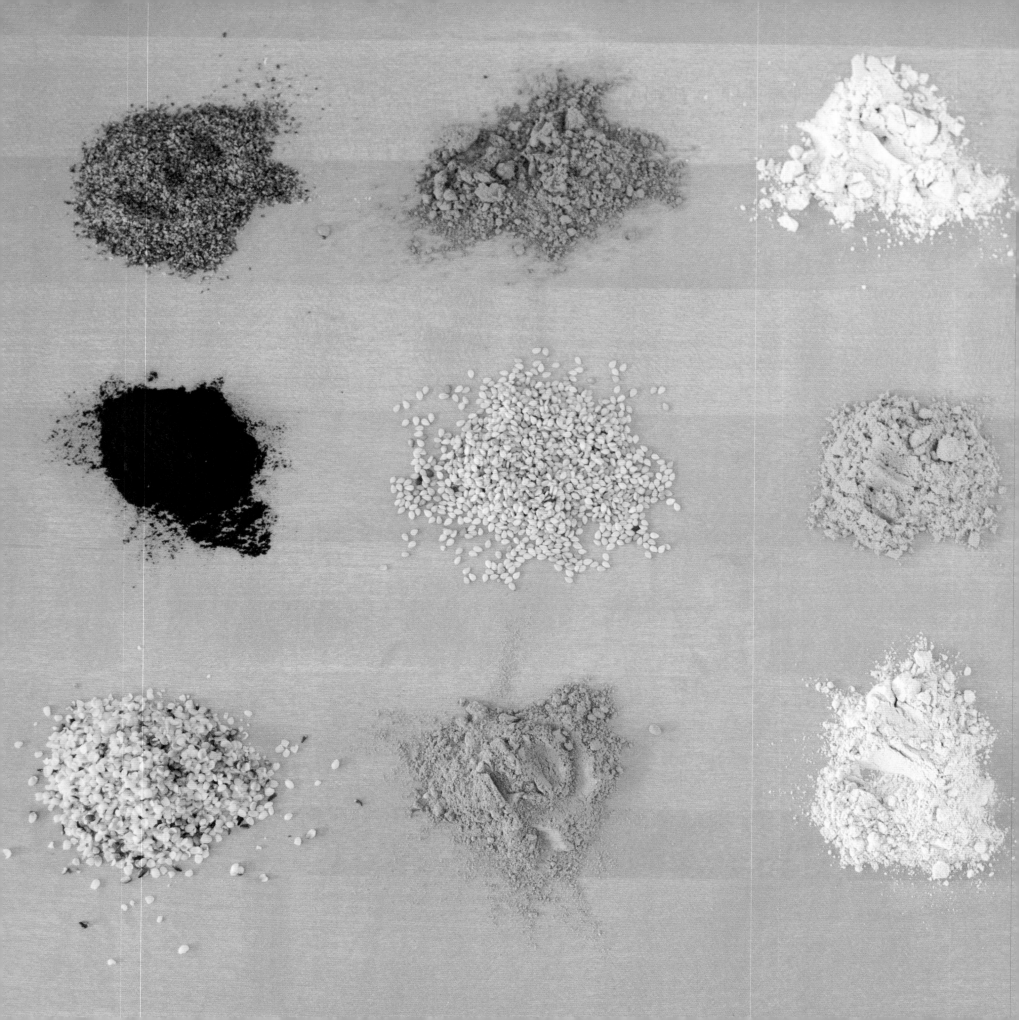

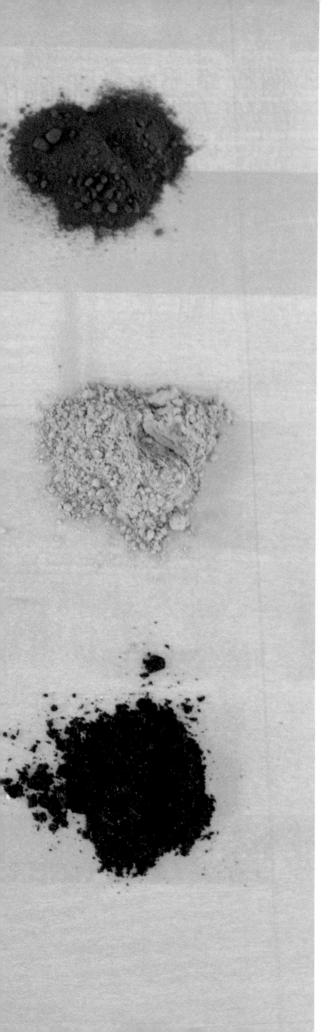

THE GOLDEN SUPERFOODS GROUP

All are used in our smoothies and soups

Ahiflower Oil

Matcha

Turmeric

Ginger

Mila Chia Seeds

E3Live Aqua Botanical Algae

Goji Berries

Hemp Seeds

Maca

Wheatgrass

Mulberries

Cacao

Spirulina

Chlorella

Medicinal Mushrooms

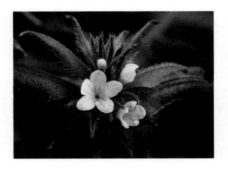

AHIFLOWER® OIL

Ahiflower oil is a nutritional powerhouse that offers an unparalleled combination of essential omega-3, -6 and -9 fatty acids. Unlike fish and flax, Ahiflower contains GLA, an omega-6 associated with skin health, hormonal balance and inflammation reduction. Ahiflower oil is clinically proven to be 300 to 400 percent more effective in omega-3 EPA conversion than flaxseed oil. Ahiflower oil also has a clean taste and aroma and no 'yuck factor' – no fishy burps or after taste. While a month's supply of typical Peruvian fish oil takes about 60 fish out of the ocean, a month's supply of Ahiflower oil only takes about 60 square feet of sustainably managed, non-GMO Ahiflower seed crop to grow year after year.[18]

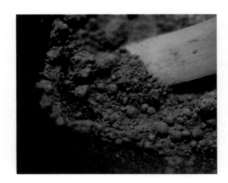

MATCHA

Matcha is a ground green tea from Japan that comes from the same plant most tea comes from, *Camellia sinesis*. High-quality matcha should have an electric green color, a smooth, savory and slightly sweet note to it, with a long finish. It helps to cleanse and detoxify the body, lowers blood pressure, enhances brain function, helps improve memory, decreases bad cholesterol, helps stabilize blood sugar levels and can increase thermogenesis, which is the body's own rate of burning calories – the benefits really go on and on! The high amount of EGCG (epigallocatechin gallate) content helps to neutralize bacterial toxins, induces apoptosis (a term used to describe the normal and constant process of cell death in living organisms) and helps to stop progress and metastasis of cancer cells. It is rich in phytonutrients, antioxidants, vitamins and minerals and contains 20 times more antioxidant power than blueberries, pomegranates or goji berries.[19]

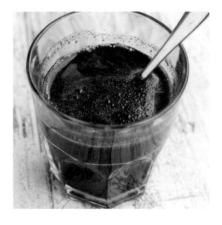

E3LIVE AQUA BOTANICAL ALGAE

E3Live is a trademarked brand of organic, wild-harvested algae from upper Klamath Lake, Oregon, and is considered one of nature's most beneficial superfoods. Nutritionally, it is packed with over 65 vitamins, minerals, amino acids, essential fatty acids and a powerful source of chlorophyll. It directly supports the immune, endocrine, nervous, gastrointestinal and cardiovascular systems.[20]

TURMERIC

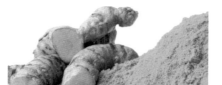

Turmeric is a golden root with an endless array of health benefits. It possesses a potent nutrient called curcumin, which is responsible for its vibrant orange color. It is considered a spice with a peppery flavor and is a popular ingredient in curries. It's known to be an incredible anti-inflammatory and a remedy to many illnesses. The spice has been used for more than 5,000 years, and to this day it plays an important role in traditional cultures throughout the Eastern world. In just a couple of tablespoons of ground turmeric, you will get almost 20 percent of your daily manganese requirements, 10 percent of iron, five percent of vitamin B and around three percent of potassium, copper and fiber. It is an anticoagulant, and appears to prevent platelet stickiness, which helps with the prevention of heart disease and strokes. It is a powerful antioxidant that is very effective in fighting free radicals, which in turn protects your skin, eyes and hair.[21]

GINGER

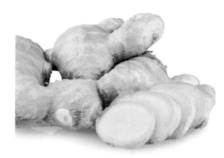

Ginger is one of the world's greatest medicines and has been used in India and China since 5000 BC. This root contains gingerol, an active constituent that is responsible for its spicy taste and stimulating anti-cancer properties. Ginger has vitamins B3, B6, C, E, folic acid, calcium, copper, iron, magnesium, manganese, phosphorus, potassium, selenium and zinc. Its volatile oil works wonders on our digestive system by protecting against indigestion and premature aging and by helping with overall absorption of valuable nutrients. The root helps regulate blood sugar levels by stimulating the pancreas cells and lowering cholesterol levels. Ginger is essential for a healthy immune system. It reduces pain and body inflammation, relieves cramping, peptic ulcers, allergies and asthma, and is used to treat joint and swelling problems.

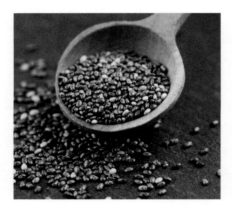

MILA* CHIA SEEDS

Chia is an edible seed that comes from the desert plant *Salvia hispanica L.*, which is grown in Mexico and dates back to Mayan and Aztec cultures. 'Chia' means strength, and folklore has it that these cultures used the tiny black and white seeds as an energy booster. Chia seed has one of the highest naturally occurring amounts of omega-3 fatty acids of any plant source. Chia contains ALA, the short-chain omega-3, which differs from the long-chain omega-3s, DHA and EPA (eicosapentaenoic acid and docosahexaenoic acid respectively), found in fish and algae oils. Chia is a complete protein food that can be absorbed by the body and provides a mix of omega-3 fatty acids and fiber, which has been shown to lower cholesterol and reduce the risk of coronary heart disease. Additionally, the seed contains high levels of antioxidants, phytonutrients and calcium.[22]

*Note: Not all chia has a complete nutritional content. Mila is the only blend I have found on the market that shares these important qualities. It is the only chia seed mix that is sliced, which increases the bioavailability of the nutrients, while preserving the oil. Mila is a blend of chia seeds grown within two degrees North or South of the equator, which gives this chia the highest amount of nutrients.

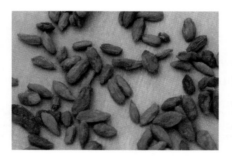

GOJI BERRIES

Known as the world's most powerful anti-aging food, goji berries are rated number one on the "oxygen radical absorbance capacity" (ORAC) scale, which measures the antioxidant level of foods. They contain eight of the nine essential amino acids that the body needs to obtain from food every day to help build protein and per ounce, organic goji berries contain even more vitamin C than oranges. As a natural source of this nutrient, goji berries boost the immune system and help your body ward off colds and infection. Organic goji berries are also extremely rich in vitamin A, which helps protect the eye's cornea and supports good vision.

HEMP SEEDS

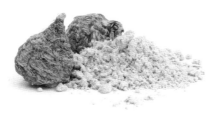

Raw organic hemp seeds out of the shell are also known as "hemp hearts" and are one of the world's most nutritious seeds. Shelled hemp seeds are 33 percent protein and packed with omega-3 fatty acids. You should eat two tablespoons or more a day of these seeds in order to receive all of their health benefits. They are a highly digestible source of plantbased protein and are a complete protein, containing all nine essential amino acids, required for our bodies to build protein. Hemp seeds contain a healthy 3-to-1 ratio of omega-6 and omega-3 fatty acids that can help control inflammation levels and prevent chronic conditions such as heart disease. Hemp hearts are also a great source of vitamin E, which acts as an antioxidant to protect cells, and iron, which wards off fatigue and boosts energy levels.[22]

MACA

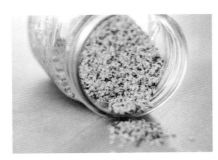

Maca (*Lepidium meyenii*) is a finicky root, similar to a turnip or radish, that only grows well in the cold, arid climates of high mountain plateaus. It is native to the Peruvian Andes, where it is still cultivated and carried to the villages below to be dried and ground into organic maca powder. Maca powder has a subtle, sweet butterscotch flavor, which makes it easy to incorporate into everyday smoothies and soups. It is a good source of B-complex vitamins and minerals such as calcium, zinc and iron. The high fiber content in maca helps stabilize blood sugar levels, increase energy and relieve stress. With seven essential amino acids, maca powder is a nearly complete source of protein.

WHEATGRASS

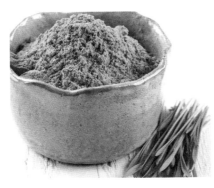

Organic wheatgrass is considered one of the most potent leafy green vegetables around. It is packed with beta-carotene, vitamin C, calcium, chlorophyll, fiber, iron and vitamin K. Wheatgrass is the sprouted shoot of wheat that contains an abundance of chlorophyll, which helps detoxify and cleanse the body while eliminating harmful toxins. Chlorophyll also has an alkalizing effect on the body and balances our pH levels. This alkalizing process also helps deliver oxygen to cells, which boosts energy. By weight, wheatgrass is approximately 85 percent pure plant protein and is made up of more than 20 amino acids.

MULBERRIES

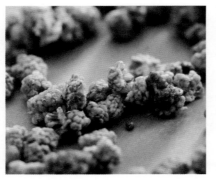

Snacking on organic mulberries is a healthy habit that you can enjoy every day. Rich in soluble fiber, organic sun dried mulberries can help lower cholesterol levels and regulate blood sugar, helping to improve the symptoms of conditions such as heart disease and diabetes. These long but smaller super berries also provide impressive levels of vitamin C and iron that boost your immune system and energy levels. They are a rare source of antioxidants known as anthocyanins, which have anti-inflammatory and possible anti-cancer effects. Studies also indicate that another antioxidant found in mulberries, known as resveratrol, has been associated with lowering blood pressure and reducing the risk for heart disease. Mulberries are also high in protein and calcium.

CACAO

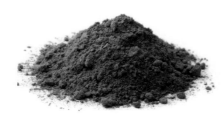

Organic raw cacao powder is created by taking the nibs and then cold-pressing the oil out. When the oil is removed from the nibs, what results is a dense, nutritionally packed dry mass, which is then ground into fine powder using no heat, which ensures maximum potency results. The protective flavonoids in organic cacao powder can protect cells against damage by free radicals. Researchers at Cornell University found that a cup of cocoa contains nearly twice the antioxidants present in a glass of red wine, up to three times the antioxidants found in a cup of green tea, and five times the concentration in a cup of black tea. These findings are published in the *Journal of Agriculture and Food Chemistry*. Organic cacao powder is also rich in flavonoids which can support heart health as well as being a natural mood booster by stimulating the release of endorphins and serotonin in the brain. Cacao is one of the richest food sources of magnesium, which aids over 300 chemical reactions in the body. It supports everything from cardiovascular function to bone health. A one-ounce serving of cacao powder contains over 30 percent of the daily value for magnesium.

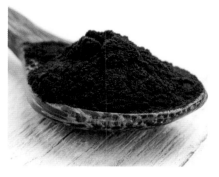

SPIRULINA

Spirulina is a type of blue-green algae found in most lakes and ponds. It's a protein and mineral powerhouse that's loaded with vitamins A through E, iron, potassium, calcium, zinc and antioxidants. It's considered a complete protein, containing an ideal balance of all nine essential amino acids. A one-ounce serving of spirulina contains over 30 percent of the daily value for protein. Spirulina's protein is 85 to 95 percent digestible, a higher percentage than that of even red meat or soy. Spirulina's antioxidant concentration is four times that of blueberries. Antioxidants protect our cells from the damaging oxidative effects of free radicals.

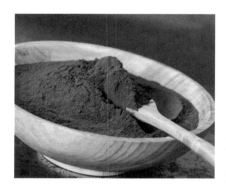

CHLORELLA

Organic chlorella (*Chlorella pyrenoidosa*) is an emerald green, single-celled freshwater algae that grows naturally in lakes and ponds. It is a true superfood, packed with nearly 10 times the healthy chlorophyll of similar greens such as wheatgrass, barley and alfalfa. Organic chlorella powder is at least 60 percent crude protein and is also a complete protein, meaning it contains a full balance of essential amino acids. It contains iron, calcium, magnesium, potassium, vitamins A, B12, C and E. If you're looking for a natural way to cleanse and detoxify, adding a small amount of this potent powder to your daily diet is an easy, gentle way to start. Organic chlorella algae is thought to bind with heavy metals, synthetic chemicals and other toxins, helping to expel them from the body. It can also promote a healthy balance of natural bacteria in the gastrointestinal tract, which can help soothe ulcers, constipation and other intestinal issues. I recommend using the best organic chlorella, as you want the powder to have mechanically cracked cell walls to ensure the bioavailability of its complete protein, vitamins and minerals.

For information on other superfoods we use, visit *projectyoubewell.com.*

MEDICINAL MUSHROOMS

For thousands of years, mushrooms have been used to
help feed people around the world, but they do more than
just keep us alive. They also can help promote health by
reducing inflammation, boosting our overall immunity and
just giving our bodies more energy. The trick is knowing
and finding which mushrooms you can eat and how to use
them wisely in your everyday diet. I will show you just
that, by sharing both smoothie and soup recipes using all
of these amazing medicinal mushrooms.

Shiitake, maitaki and cremini mushrooms are easy to find fresh in most markets and I use these three types fresh when I make my smoothies and soups. However, when I want to really bring the recipe up to superfood status I use mushroom mycelial extract powders. Mycelial extract powders are essentially a mushroom superfood, primarily consisting of the mycelium (white vegetable growth) of each mushroom species. Mycelium-based extract powders are generally considered to be more potent than powders derived solely from mushroom caps.

Cordyceps have been used to treat a range of health conditions, from type 2 diabetes to severe asthma. Now experts are focusing on the potential of cordyceps to improve kidney function in patients undergoing a kidney transplant. Athletes covet these mushrooms, as they are known for boosting your endurance, vitality and post workout recovery.

These fascinating **reishi** mushrooms are so potent because of their unique collection of organic compounds and components, which include triterpenes, alkaloids, sterols, and various essential polysaccharides. They have a tough texture and quite a bitter taste and are really considered to be solely for medicinal use. They have been called the mushroom of immortality and have many antibacterial and antiviral properties, making it a great choice for fighting off nasty colds or infections.

Shiitake mushrooms help boost the body's energy levels, improve immunity, lower cholesterol and even fight cancer. Research published by the *Journal of Clinical Oncology* suggests eating uber-rich shiitake mushrooms consistently can help slow the development of some types of cancer cells.[23]

Maitake is a meaty mushroom widely known by chefs as the dancing culinary mushroom. Maitake is believed to have a significant effect on slowing down the growth and development of cancer cells (according to limited clinical trials). They have also been used to help control diabetes, lower cholesterol and stabilize blood pressure.

Lion's Mane mushrooms actually look like a lion's mane! This type of mushroom is believed to boost memory, improve cognitive functionality and boost overall brain function. This mushroom is also known to boost the strength of the body's immune system.

Turkey Tail mushrooms are one of the most studied mushrooms in the world because researchers have been investigating its cancer-fighting properties. In Japan, the turkey tail mushroom has been used in cancer treatment plans for more than three decades.

Chaga mushrooms are known to help boost the immune system, aid in inflammation and fight viruses. They have strong antifungal and anti-tumor properties and contain a strong antioxidant, called superoxide dismutase (SOD). They also contain minerals such as zinc and geranium and a good dose of vitamin D.

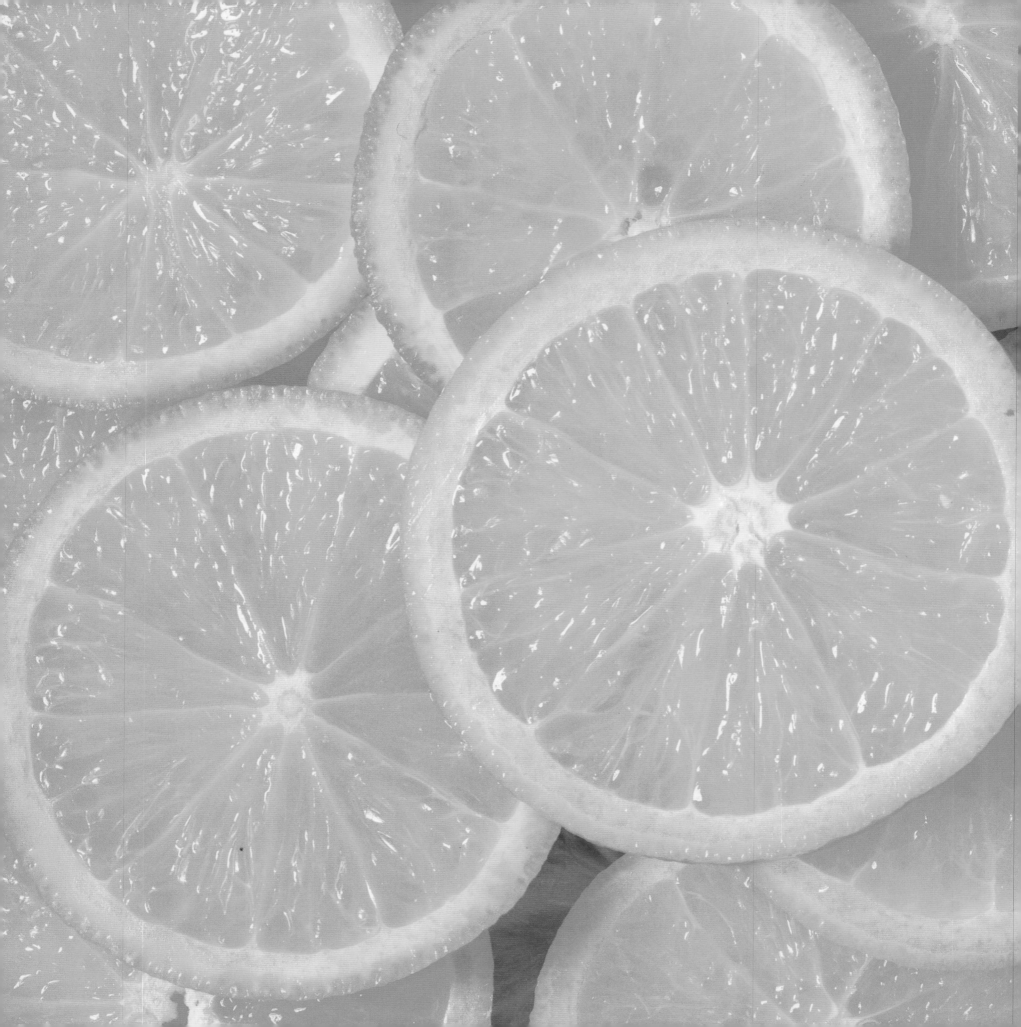

Chapter 6

WHAT'S IN COMMON SUPERFOODS?

While my Australian "Fab Four" and "Golden" superfoods are exotic, here I introduce more common superfoods that you can find at your local market, as well as the vitamins, minerals and other nutritional elements they contain. I use all of these superfoods in my smoothies and soups.

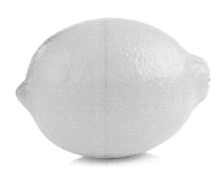

LEMONS

Vitamins B3, B5, B6, C, E, beta carotene, biotin, folic acid, calcium, copper, iodine, iron, magnesium, manganese, phosphorus, potassium, selenium, zinc, flavonoids, limonene

Lemons are powerhouses of antioxidant vitamin C, which boosts our immune system, aids in the healing of wounds and strengthens the walls of blood capillaries. The high level of vitamin C means that they are vital for healthy skin and gums. They are a good source of flavonoids, such as quercetin, which gives the big boost for the effects of vitamin C. Lemons are also a liver stimulant and can be used for detoxification. Lemons contain limonene, a chemical that has been shown to slow the growth of cancer.

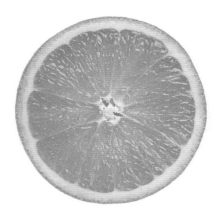

ORANGES

Vitamins A, B1, B3, B5, C, E and K, beta carotene, folic acid, calcium, iodine, magnesium, phosphorus, potassium, selenium, zinc, limonene, hesperidin, fiber

Oranges are a top source of vitamin C, which is important for building immunity and fighting viruses. They are helpful in reducing post-exercise muscle soreness and combating colds, flu and respiratory ailments such as asthma. Oranges have been found to help reduce the risk of stomach ulcers and kidney stones. They contain beta-sitosterol, a plant sterol that helps prevent tumor formation. Oranges are high in fiber and very rich in vitamin B5, which stimulates the body's immune response. Oranges, abundant in vitamins and minerals, help maintain healthy youthful skin.

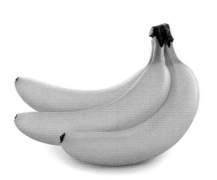

BANANAS

Vitamins B2, B3, B6, C and K, beta-carotene, biotin, folic acid, calcium, iodine, iron, magnesium, manganese, phosphorus, potassium, selenium, zinc, fiber, carbohydrate, tryptophan

Bananas are the go-to food when you're "on the run". They provide a potent mix of vitamins, minerals and carbohydrates and contain tryptophan, which the body converts to serotonin to ease depression and promote peaceful sleep. Bananas contain high levels of B vitamins, including B5, which boosts the immune system, and B6, which improves the body's ability to clear away waste matter, reduce fatigue and premenstrual symptoms. Bananas are also high in potassium, which regulates body fluids and nerve function. Bananas contain the ideal carbohydrate combination to replace muscle glycogen before or during exercise, making them a very valuable food for athletes.

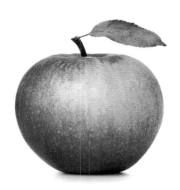

APPLES

Vitamins B3, C, E and K, beta-carotene, biotin, folic acid, calcium, chromium, iron, magnesium, manganese, phosphorus, potassium, zinc, malic acid, quercetin, flavonoids, fiber

An apple a day does keep the doctor away! Apples have many health benefits including improved digestion and detoxification. Apples are also rich in soluble and insoluble fiber, both of which help food to pass through the digestive system at a healthy pace. These fibers pick up toxic waste, such as heavy metals and cholesterol, which are safely excreted with the help of soluble fiber and pectin.

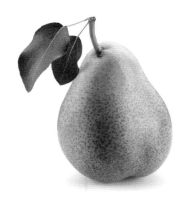

PEARS

Vitamins B3, C, E and K, beta carotene, biotin, folic acid, calcium, copper, iodine, iron, magnesium, phosphorus, potassium, zinc, fiber

Pears have both soluble and insoluble fiber but it contains a higher amount of insoluble fiber, which works like tiny scrubbing brushes in the colon to promote good digestion. The insoluble fiber also helps to eliminate cholesterol from the body. The antioxidant vitamin C and folic acid content in pears also boost immunity and fight off infections.

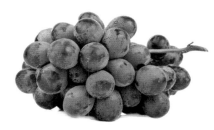

GRAPES

Vitamins B1, B3, B6, C and K, beta carotene, biotin, folic acid, calcium, copper, iodine, iron, magnesium, manganese, phosphorus, potassium, selenium, zinc, anthocyanins, ellagic acid, flavonoids, quercetin and fiber

Grapes are one of those powerful fruits that can prevent and treat many age-related conditions, from anemia and fatigue to arthritis, varicose veins and rheumatism. They are very rich in minerals – selenium in particular, which is great for skin and helps to keep fine lines and wrinkles at bay. Grapes are full of antioxidants, including astringent tannins, flavonoids and anthocyanins, which help prevent bad LDL cholesterol from oxidizing. Grapes contain cancer-preventing ellagic acid and resveratrol.

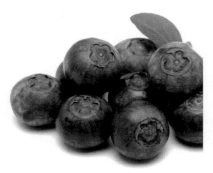

BLUEBERRIES

Vitamins B2, B3, B5, C, E and K, beta carotene, folic acid, calcium, iron, magnesium, manganese, phosphorus, potassium, selenium, zinc, flavonoids, ellagic acid, tannins

Blueberries are one of the strongest super fruits that protect our cells from free radical damage and aging. These berries get their deep blue color from anthocyanins, which are potent antioxidants that combat cell damage, improve circulation and help protect against heart problems. The antioxidant ellagic acid and the compound resveratrol, both found in blueberries, have been shown to help prevent the growth of cancer. Lastly, proanthocyanidins (a type of flavonoids contained in blueberries) increase the potency of vitamin C, which helps support collagen for skin elasticity.

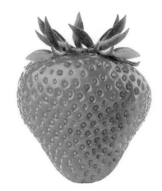

STRAWBERRIES

Vitamins B2, B3, B5, B6, C and K, folic acid, copper, iron, magnesium, manganese, iodine, potassium, flavonoids, ellagic acid and omega 3 fatty acids

Strawberries are packed with vitamin C, which is essential for manufacturing collagen, a protein that helps to maintain the structure of the skin by keeping it elastic and young-looking. Collagen also helps in healing wounds. These berries contain ellagic acid, a phytochemical that's been shown to help fight cancer and destroy some of the toxins in our body. Their B vitamins help support the nervous system, while their high iron content makes them therapeutic for fatigue.

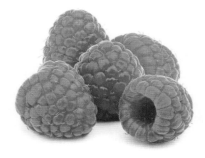

RASPBERRIES

Vitamins B2, B3, B5, C and K, beta-carotene, biotin, folic acid, calcium, copper, iodine, iron, magnesium, manganese, phosphorus, potassium, selenium, zinc, ellagic acid

Raspberries are great for detoxing the body and keeping blood-sugar levels steady. They aid in keeping cholesterol low and are high in anthocyanins, which are powerful antioxidants that help our bodies produce cells that fight off free radicals. The anthocyanins in raspberries contain anti-inflammatory properties which help ease joint pain and arthritis. Raspberries contain high levels of vitamin C which help with infections and body immunity. These wonder fruits contain ellagic acid, which is anti-carcinogenic and responsible for preventing adverse cellular changes.

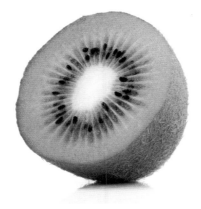

KIWI FRUITS

Vitamins B3, B5, B6, C and E, beta carotene, biotin, folic acid, lutein, calcium, copper, iodine, iron, magnesium, manganese, phosphorus, potassium, selenium, zinc

The immunity-boosting kiwi fruits contains more vitamin C than oranges. Just one fruit has 120 percent of an adult's daily recommended intake. Vitamin C not only wards off colds but also protects the body from all kinds of infections and inflammation. Kiwi fruits are also loaded with lutein, a carotenoid that, together with vitamins C and E, is fantastic for preserving youthful skin and protecting vision. Kiwi fruits are high in potassium which helps prevent high blood pressure and insomnia.

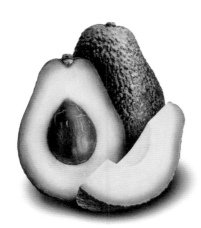

AVOCADOS

Vitamins B1, B2, B3, B5, B6, C, E, K, biotin, carotenoids, folic acid, calcium, copper, iodine, iron, magnesium, manganese, phosphorus, potassium, zinc, beta-sitosterol, glutathione, omega 3, 6 and 9 fatty acids

The avocado, which is a type of pear, is the richest fruit source of moisturizing monounsaturated fatty acid, which does wonders for your skin and hair. The omega-9 fats help balance the moisture levels in the epidermal layer of the skin and keep the skin supple. The oleic acid present in avocados helps reduce facial irritations and aids in the regeneration of skin cells that have been damaged. Another beneficial fat in avocados, lecithin, plays a big role in brain function. This creamy delicious fruit has mega amounts of vitamin E, which is an important antioxidant that neutralizes the damaging effects of toxins and helps boost resistance against infections.

For information on other common superfoods we use, visit *projectyoubewell.com.*

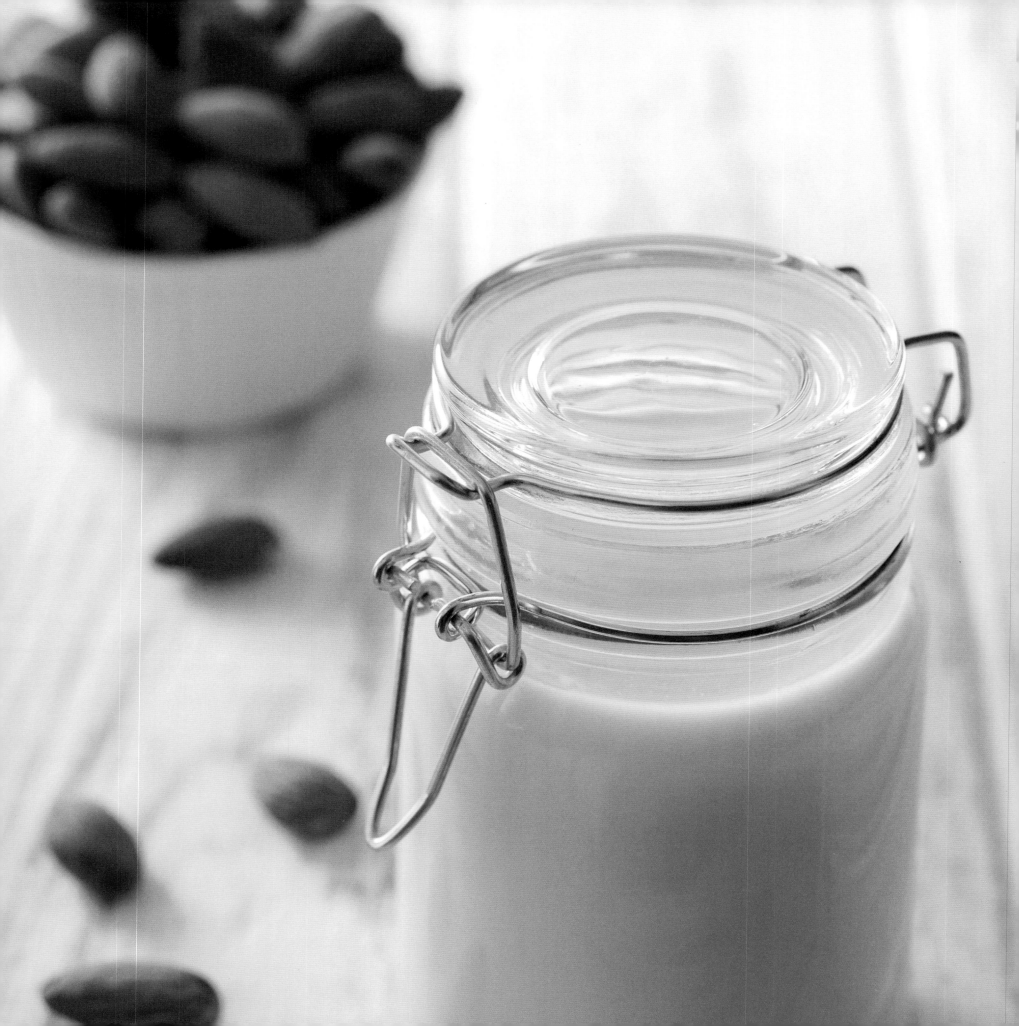

HOMEMADE NUTMILKS

Homemade nutmilks are tasty, healthy and easy to make. You soak the raw nuts or seeds in water and blend with one and a half teaspoons of vanilla extract, a dash of sea salt, raw cacao or cinnamon (see soaking times and ratios below). The amount of soaking water used does not matter as long as the nuts and seeds are covered. Soak then rinse the nuts in plenty of cold water. It's important when making almond milk to discard the soaking water because it contains phytic acid, which inhibits the body's ability to absorb nutrients. After washing, combine almonds or other varieties with clean water into a blender and blend for two minutes.

All my nutmilks have a slightly mild sweet taste and a beautiful creamy texture. There are many new nutmilk varieties out on the market, but I prefer to make mine, as they are fresher than packaged milks and have zero preservatives. Homemade nutmilks usually last about three to four days in the refrigerator, so only make as much as you really need.

INSTRUCTIONS FOR MAKING THE TASTIEST NUTMILKS

1. Soak nuts and seeds in a glass bowl or large glass Mason jar in clean water. Make sure all nuts or seeds are covered completely (see soaking times below). Coconut meat does not need to be soaked.
2. Strain out all soaking water and rinse nuts or seeds with fresh water.
3. Put nuts, seeds or coconut meat along with clean water (see chart) into blender. Blend until completely smooth and creamy. For coconut milk use the coconut's water for a sweeter blend or clean water for a less sweet coconut milk.
4. Pour milk into nut bag or cheese cloth and strain out nut and seed meal from milk. For coconut milk you can skip this step.

NUT/SEED MILK CHART:

NUT/SEED	QUANTITY	WATER	SOAK TIME
ALMONDS	1 cup	2 cups	6+ hours
CASHEWS	1 cup	2 cups	2+ hours
HEMP SEEDS	½ cup	1¼ cups	1-2 hours
SUNFLOWER SEEDS	½ cup	1¼ cups	2+ hours
PUMPKIN SEEDS	½ cup	1½ cups	2+ hours
RAW COCONUT	1 young Thai coconut	1½ cups	None

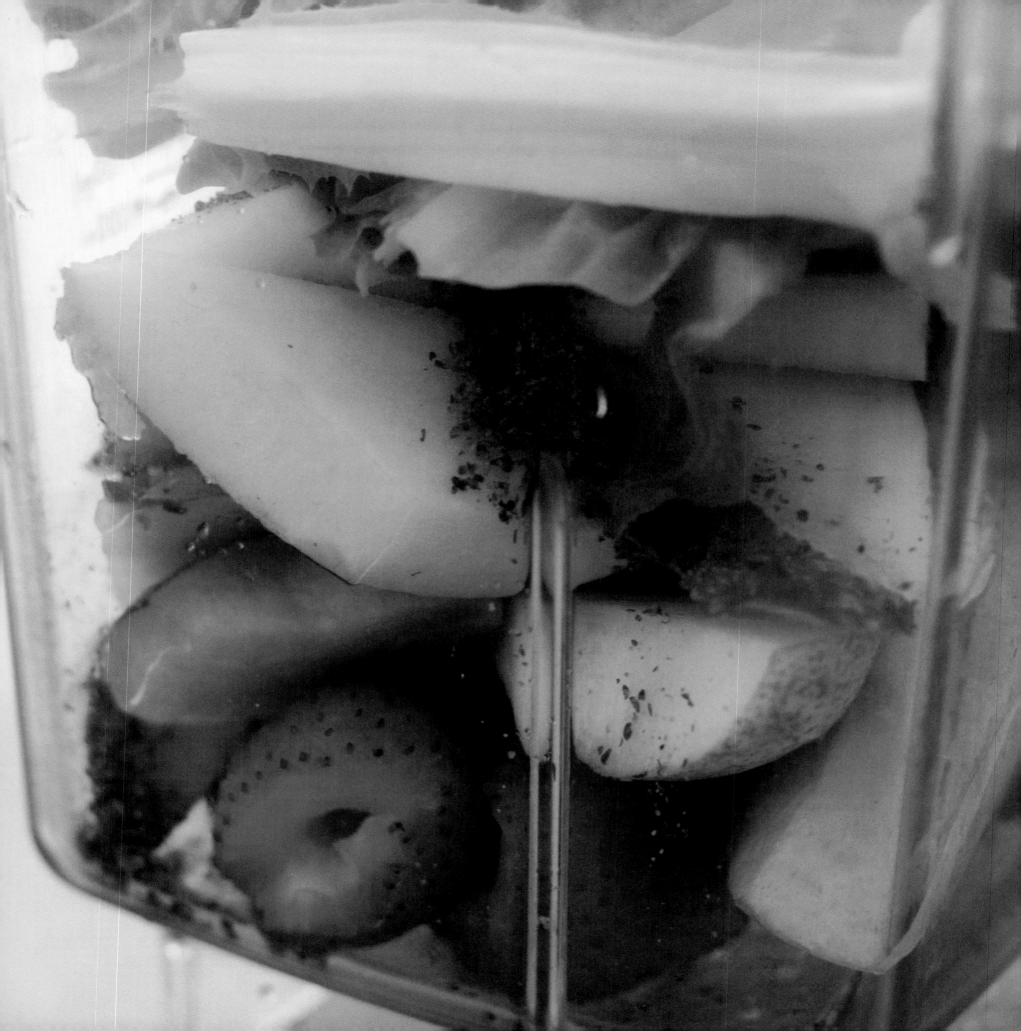

Chapter 7

SUPERFOOD SMOOTHIE & PUDDING RECIPES

If you think the strawberry banana smoothie you drink every morning is helping you lose weight and live a healthier life, think again. Most smoothies are ridiculously high in sugar – some packing more sugar than you'd find in two cans of Coke! Even natural sugars found in fruits and honey can send your blood-sugar levels sky high.

The good news is that you can make nutritious and delicious smoothies packed with vitamin-, mineral- and antioxidant-rich superfoods. My smoothies will boost your energy and immunity, while keeping your blood sugar levels stable. Every ingredient I use is carefully mixed for optimal taste and health benefits, but all of my recipes can be tweaked to your specific palette.

SMOOTHIE DIRECTIONS

With all smoothies, add heavier items in blender first, followed by lighter items and then liquids. Add a handful of ice at the end. It's that easy.

A NOTE ON SWEETENERS

I typically do not use any added sweeteners in my smoothies except for the raw fruits and vegetables themselves. My smoothies are plenty sweet on their own. For those of you who would like to sweeten up your smoothies a little more, you can use a pinch of stevia, NuStevia or a small amount of raw unrefined coconut crystals. Overall, I try to keep my smoothies low on the glycemic index. Natural sweeteners such as honey, agave nectar, maple and date syrup can be used occasionally in micro amounts, but they are still high on the glycemic index and when paired with fruit could make a smoothie much too sweet for your body. Corn syrup, cane sugar and evaporated cane juice should never be used to sweeten food.

High speed blender recommendations, see Resources.

For more delicious smoothie recipes visit my website, *projectyoubewell.com*

BANANA ALMOND BUTTER CHOCOLATE SMOOTHIE

Serves 2

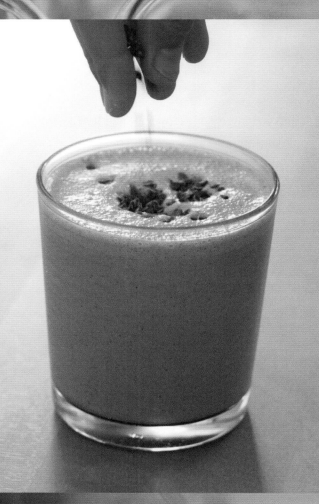

1 banana, peeled

2 tablespoons raw almond butter

1 tablespoon raw cacao powder

1 tablespoon raw hemp seeds

1 tablespoon Mila chia seeds

1 tablespoon sesame seeds

2 large leaves kale

1 cup homemade (or unsweetened store-bought) almond milk

½ teaspoon Ahiflower oil

Handful cacao nibs (optional)

Handful ice (optional)

BLUEBERRY MINT SMOOTHIE

Serves 2

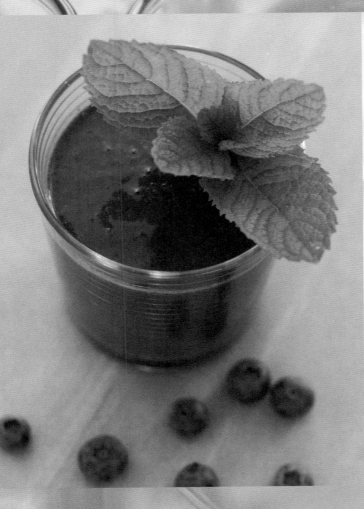

1 cup fresh or frozen blueberries

1 cup romaine lettuce

4 fresh (or dried) shiitake mushrooms

1 banana, peeled

¼ cup kefir yogurt, or
1 tablespoon prebiotic powder
(see Resources on where to buy)

2 large sprigs mint

1 cup unsweetened almond milk

4 medjool dates

½ cup filtered (or spring) water

1 tablespoon raw cacao powder

½ teaspoon Ahiflower oil

½ teaspoon riberry powder (optional)

Handful ice (optional)

BLUEBERRY YAM SMOOTHIE

Serves 2

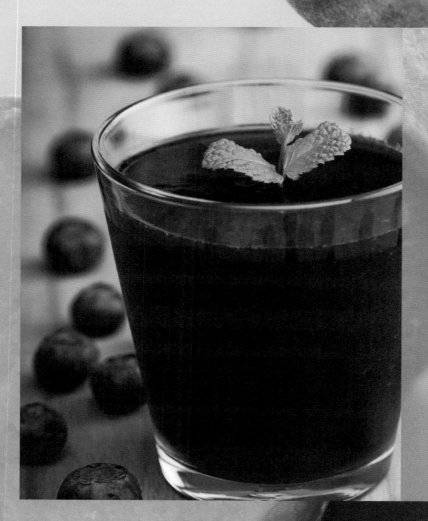

1 cup fresh blueberries (use frozen if fresh not available)

½ teaspoon spirulina/chlorella powder mix
(I combine equal amounts of each powder in
a large jar to use together)

1 tablespoon raw hemp seeds

½ chunk purple Okinawan sweet potato (or yam),
baked, skin removed and halved

½ cup unsweetened kefir yogurt, or 1 tablespoon
prebiotic powder (see Resources on where to buy)

½ peach, roughly chopped

1½ bananas, peeled

1 tablespoon Mila chia seeds

½ teaspoon Ahiflower oil

½ teaspoon davidson plum powder

Handful ice (optional)

Mint, to garnish

BLUEBERRY SHIITAKE SMOOTHIE

Serves 2

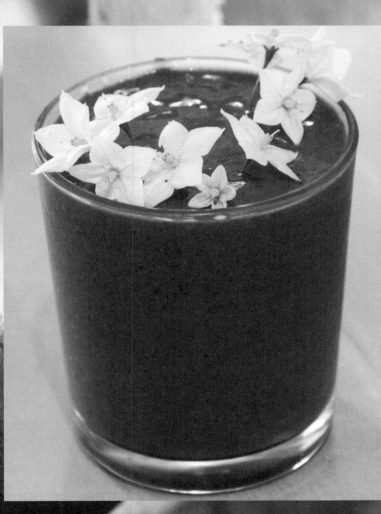

4 dried shiitake mushrooms

1½ cups fresh (or frozen) blueberries

1 banana, peeled

1 tablespoon raw hemp seeds

1 tablespoon unhulled sesame seeds

1 tablespoon Mila chia seeds

1 knob fresh turmeric

½ inch knob fresh ginger

½ cup super greens powder

1 cup Harmless Harvest coconut water

1 cup filtered (or spring) water

½ teaspoon Ahiflower oil

½ teaspoon davidson plum powder (optional)

Handful ice (optional)

POMEGRANATE TANGERINE SMOOTHIE

Serves 2

Seeds of 1 pomegranate, rinsed

1 tangerine, peeled

1 cup frozen mango, or 1 large mango, roughly chopped

½ teaspoon kakadu plum powder

½ sweet potato

1 cup homemade (or unsweetened store-bought) almond milk

½ cup filtered (or spring) water

1 tablespoon Mila chia seed

½ teaspoon Ahiflower oil

Handful ice (optional)

MATCHA KIWI SMOOTHIE

Serves 2

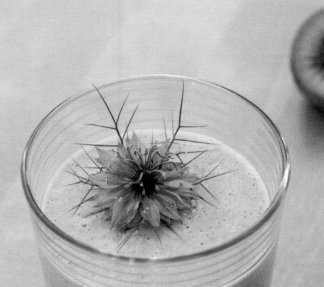

3 kiwifruits, roughly chopped

½ teaspoon kakadu plum powder

1 cup raw spinach

1 cup fresh dino kale

1 cup homemade (or unsweetened store-bought) almond milk

¾ cup filtered (or spring) water

1 tablespoon flax, ground

1 teaspoon organic matcha green tea powder

1 tablespoon almond meal

Juice of 1 tangerine

½ teaspoon Ahiflower oil

Handful ice (optional)

MACADAMIA NUTTY BANANA SMOOTHIE

Serves 2

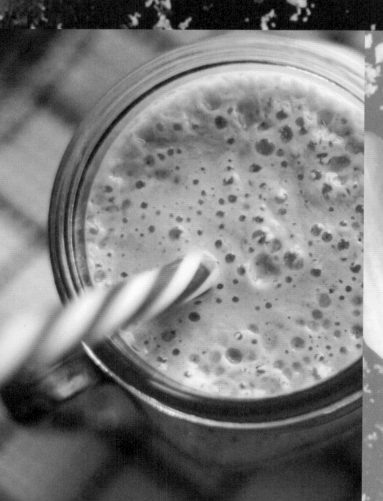

2 bananas, peeled

2½ tablespoons raw almond butter

2 tablespoons Mila chia seeds

1½ cups homemade (or unsweetened store-bought) macadamia milk

2 tablespoons low-fat plain kefir
or prebiotic powder (see Resources on where to buy)

MINTY CHOCOLATE CACAO SMOOTHIE

Serves 2

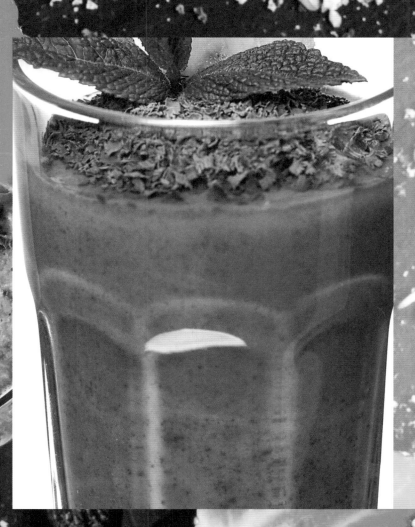

1 cup homemade (or unsweetened store-bought) almond milk

1½ cups romaine lettuce

½ cup fresh spinach

2 sprigs fresh mint (handpicked if possible)

2 tablespoons raw almond butter

½ cup store-bought hazelnut milk

1 tablespoon raw cacao

1 tablespoon raw hemp seed

1 banana, peeled

1 tablespoon Mila chia seeds

½ teaspoon Ahiflower oil

Handful ice (optional)

Handful cacao nibs (optional)

PEAR BOK CHOY SMOOTHIE

Serves 2

2½ cups fresh pears

1 tablespoon Mila chia seeds

1½ cups Harmless Harvest coconut water

½ cup low-fat kefir yogurt or prebiotic powder
(see Resources on where to buy)

4–5 fresh stalks bok choy

½ teaspoon Ahiflower oil

Handful ice (optional)

SPICY MANGO STRAWBERRY SMOOTHIE

Serves 2

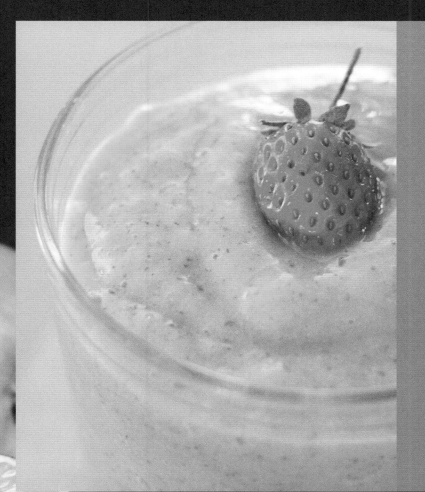

1 fresh mango, roughly chopped

1½ cups strawberries

½ teaspoon kakadu plum powder

½ teaspoon red pepper flakes

1 container GoodBelly Big Shot 50 Probiotic Drink

1 cup spinach

1 tablespoon raw hemp seeds

1 cup Harmless Harvest coconut water

1 cup filtered (or spring) water

½ teaspoon Ahiflower oil

Handful cashews

Handful ice (optional)

LEMON SPINACH MINT SMOOTHIE

Serves 2

1 banana, peeled

1 apple (pink lady if in season), sliced with skin on

1 container GoodBelly Big Shot 50 Probiotic Drink

2-inch cube organic sprouted tofu

1 cup filtered (or spring) water

3 sprigs fresh mint

1 lemon, slightly skinned (leave some of the peel on)

1 tablespoon maca powder

1 cup fresh spinach

½ teaspoon Ahiflower oil

Handful ice (optional)

TART RASPBERRY CHERRY SMOOTHIE

Serves 2

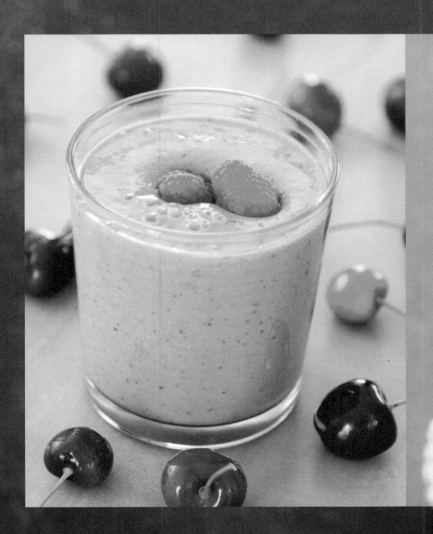

2-inch piece butternut squash, cooked

1 cup raspberries

½ teaspoon riberry powder

½ cup low-fat kefir or prebiotic powder
(see Resources on where to buy)

1 cup filtered (or spring) water

1 tablespoon almond meal

1 cup super greens lettuce mix

1 teaspoon raw hemp seeds

½ cup fresh (or frozen) wild cherries, pitted

½ teaspoon Ahiflower oil

Handful ice (optional)

JARDIN SUPER GREENS SMOOTHIE

Serves 2

1 tablespoon raw hemp seeds

1 tablespoon Mila chia seeds

1 cup Harmless Harvest coconut water

1 cup filtered (or spring) water

1 stalk celery

1 cup super greens mixed lettuce

1 cup romaine lettuce

1–2 dino kale stalks

1 banana, peeled

1 cup mango

1 pear, roughly chopped

½ teaspoon spirulina/chlorella mix (optional)

½ teaspoon Ahiflower oil

Handful ice (optional)

STRAWBERRY RHUBARB SMOOTHIE

Serves 2

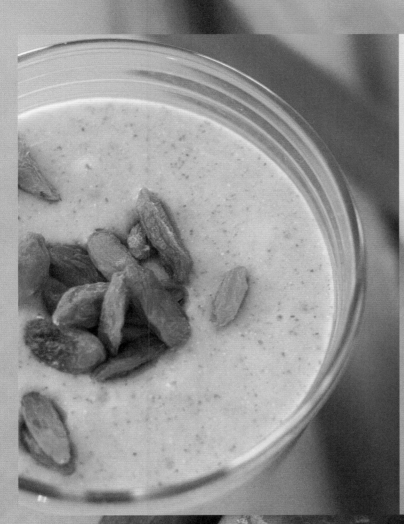

1 part strawberry and rhubarb syrup*

½ cup GoodBelly coconut probiotic drink

½ cup fresh almond or nutmilk or unsweetened almond milk from carton

1 tablespoon Mila chia seeds

1 tablespoon raw hemp seeds

1½ teaspoons sacha inchi powder

½ teaspoon kakadu plum powder

¼ tablespoon ground black pepper (optional)

½ tablespoon Ahiflower oil

Handful goji berries, to garnish

Handful ice (optional)

Heat 1½ cups strawberries with 2 stalks chopped and peeled rhubarb and 2 tablespoons maple syrup or 1 teaspoon stevia powder. Let mixture cool before adding to smoothie

CANTALOUPE SWEET YAM SMOOTHIE

Serves 2

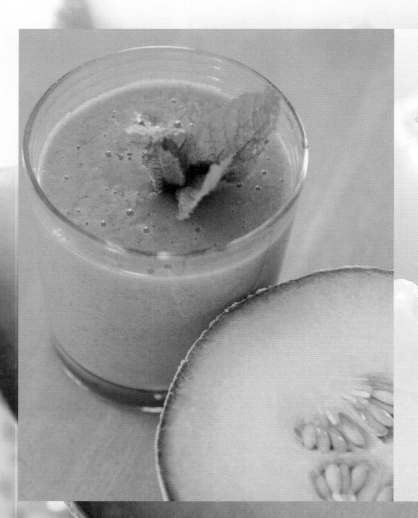

2 cups cantaloupe, finely diced

½ cup orange yam, steamed or baked

½ cup homemade cashew milk or any store-bought unsweetened nutmilk

½ cup GoodBelly Drink coconut probiotic drink

½ cup wheatgrass powder

1 sprig fresh mint

½ teaspoon Ahiflower oil

Handful ice (optional)

PINEAPPLE SMOOTHIE

Serves 2

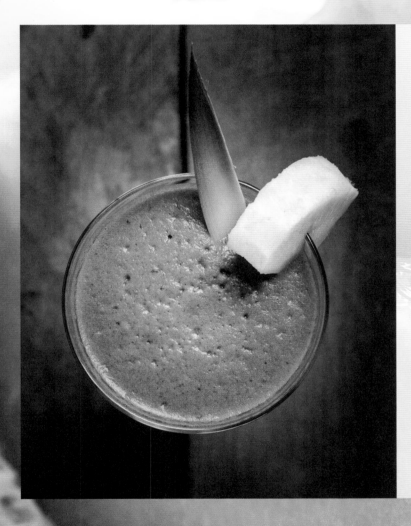

1½ cups fresh pineapple, diced

1 medium apple

1 cup fresh spinach leaves

1 banana, peeled

1½ tablespoons vanilla extract
(non-alcoholic if possible)

½ cup plain low-fat kefir yogurt

1 lemon, juice only

2 sprigs fresh mint

1 tablespoon Mila chia seed

½ cup filtered (or spring) water

½ teaspoon Ahiflower oil

Handful ice (optional)

MAMA MANGO SMOOTHIE

Serves 2

1 ripe mango or 2 cups frozen mangoes, roughly chopped

1 orange, peeled

½ teaspoon wheatgrass powder

1 cup raw coconut water or store-bought Harmless Harvest coconut water

½ teaspoon Ahiflower oil

½ cup filtered (or spring) water

1½ teaspoons maca powder

1½ teaspoons sacha inchi powder

Handful ice (optional)

KUMQUAT FIERY PEACH SMOOTHIE

Serves 2

4 small fresh kumquats, skin on, or ½ orange

1½ peaches or 1½ cups frozen peaches

1 banana, peeled

1 cup fresh (or store-bought) coconut water

1½ tablespoons Mila chia seeds

1 tablespoon flax seeds

¼ teaspoon red pepper flakes

¼ teaspoon wheatgrass

Handful ice (optional)

DRAGON FRUIT BLUEBERRY SMOOTHIE

Serves 2

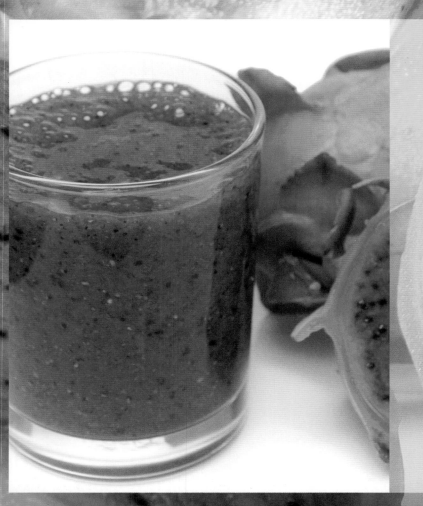

Flesh of 1 dragon fruit or 1 frozen puree pack (see Resources on where to buy)

1 cup fresh (or frozen) blueberries

1 apple, skin on

2 tablespoons raw hemp seeds

½ teaspoon wheatgrass

½ teaspoon kakadu plum powder

½ cup filtered (or spring) water

½ cup coconut (or cactus) water (see Resources on where to buy)

½ teaspoon Ahiflower oil

Handful ice (optional)

PLUM PEAR SMOOTHIE

Serves 2

3 plums, roughly chopped

2 pears, roughly chopped

1 cup fresh (or frozen) strawberries

½ teaspoon davidson plum powder

1 tablespoon raw hemp seeds

2 tablespoons Mila chia seeds

1-inch knob ginger

1½-inch knob turmeric

1 cup Harmless Harvest coconut water

1 cup filtered (or spring) water

½ teaspoon Ahiflower oil

½ teaspoon wheatgrass

Handful ice (optional)

STRAWBERRY PEACH PEAR SMOOTHIE

Serves 2

1 cup fresh (or frozen) strawberries

1 pear, roughly chopped

1 peach, roughly chopped

1 tablespoon Mila chia seeds

1½ cups romaine lettuce

1 tablespoon raw hemp seeds

1 banana (optional)

1 cup raw coconut water

2-inch cube organic Wildwood Sprouted Tofu

½ teaspoon Ahiflower oil

1 teaspoon spirulina/chlorella mix (optional)

¼ teaspoon quandong powder

Handful ice (optional)

MANGO TANGO BANANA

Serves 2

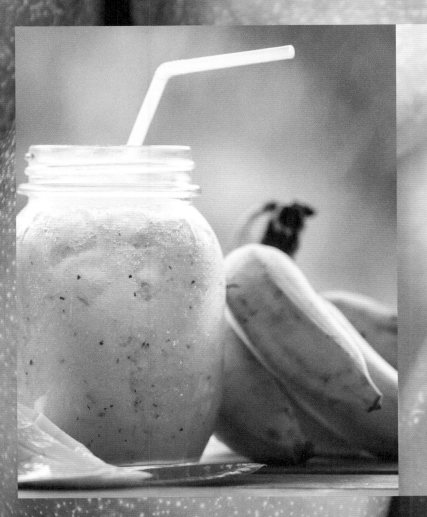

1 fresh mango, roughly chopped

1 tablespoon raw flax seeds, crushed

1 handful fresh (or frozen) strawberries

½ teaspoon riberry powder

1 banana, peeled

1 tablespoon prebiotic powder
or GoodBelly probiotic
(see Resources on where to buy)

1 cup filtered (or spring) water

1-inch knob turmeric

1-inch knob ginger

½ teaspoon Ahiflower oil

Handful ice

PINEAPPLE KALE BUTTER LETTUCE SMOOTHIE

Serves 2

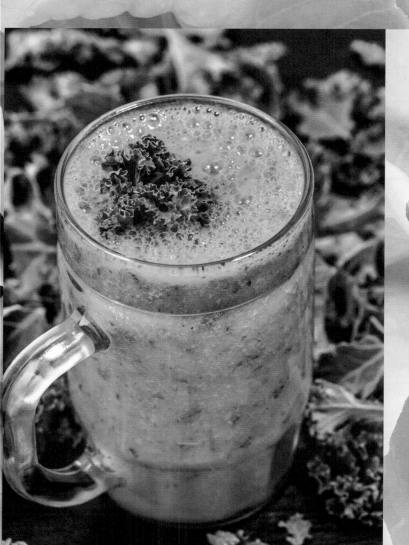

2-inch cube sprouted tofu

1 tablespoon raw hemp seeds

3 leaves kale

1½ cups butter lettuce

2 very ripe bananas, peeled

¼ cup kefir low-fat yogurt or 1 tablespoon prebiotic powder (see Resources on where to buy)

1 tablespoon Mila chia seeds

3 tablespoons E3 Live (see Resources where to buy)

1 cup Harmless Harvest coconut water

½ cup filtered (or spring) water

1 teaspoon spirulina, chlorella mix (optional)

½ teaspoon Ahiflower oil

Handful cilantro

Handful Italian flat parsley

Handful ice (optional)

ALMOND BUTTER SPINACH SMOOTHIE

Serves 2

2 cups fresh spinach

2 tablespoons almond butter

1 tablespoon raw cacao

2-inch block sprouted raw tofu

1 tablespoon raw hemp seeds

1 tablespoon raw sesame seeds

2 cups homemade (or unsweetened store-bought almond milk (see Resources on where to buy)

1 tablespoon Mila chia seeds

1 teaspoon spirulina/chlorella mix (optional)

½ teaspoon Ahiflower oil

Handful raw cashews

Handful ice (optional)

RASPBERRY SQUASH SMOOTHIE

Serves 2

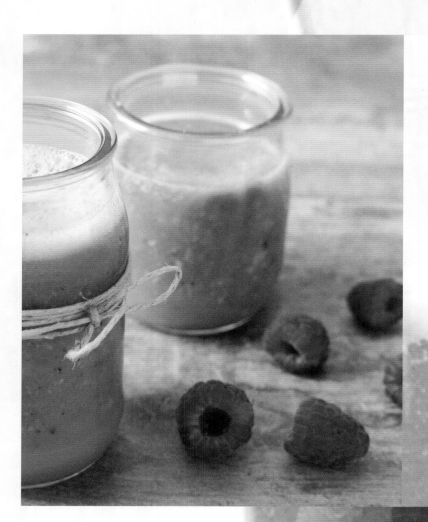

¾ cup butternut squash, cooked

2 cups frozen raspberries (use fresh if in season)

1 cup fresh spinach

1 tablespoon Mila chia seeds

1 banana, peeled

¼ cup plain low-fat kefir yogurt or prebiotic powder (see Resources on where to buy)

1½ cups Harmless Harvest coconut water

1 cup filtered (or spring) water

½ teaspoon Ahiflower oil

½ teaspoon davidson plum powder (optional)

Handful ice (optional)

POMEGRANATE MANGO SMOOTHIE

Serves 2

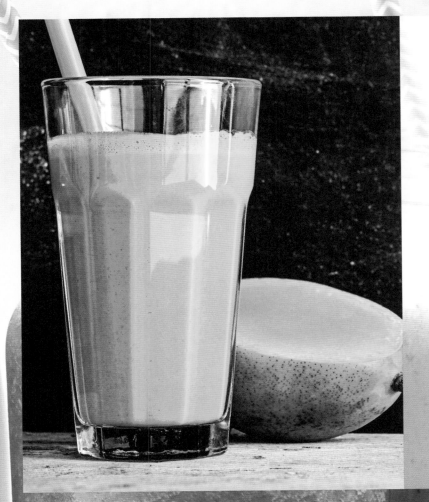

1 pomegranate, seeds only

1 cup frozen mango

1 banana, peeled

1 tablespoon Mila chia seeds

1 tablespoon flax seeds

1 cup Harmless Harvest coconut water

1½ cups filtered (or spring) water

½ teaspoon Ahiflower oil

½ teaspoon quandong powder

3 leaves dino kale (optional)

2 tablespoons raw cashews

Handful ice (optional)

GOJI BERRY SMOOTHIE

Serves 2

½ cup fresh soft goji berries

1 cup fresh strawberries

1 cup GoodBelly coconut water probiotic drink

1 tablespoon Mila chia seeds

1 teaspoon maca powder

1 tablespoon hemp seeds

½ teaspoon kakadu plum powder

1 cup raspberry kefir probiotics or GoodBelly non-dairy coconut probiotics drink

½ teaspoon Ahiflower oil

Handful ice (optional)

CACTUS PEAR STRAWBERRY SMOOTHIE

Serves 2

1 cactus pear (in season August–December)

1½ cups fresh (or frozen) strawberries

½ teaspoon kakadu plum powder

1 cup cactus water (see Resources on where to buy) or coconut water

¼ teaspoon ground pepper

¼ cup filtered (or spring) water

¼ teaspoon wheatgrass powder

1 tablespoon Mila chia Seeds

1 teaspoon maca powder

1½ teaspoons sacha inchi powder

½ teaspoon Ahiflower oil

Handful goji berries

Handful ice (optional if using fresh strawberries)

PEACHY QUANDONG GREEN SMOOTHIE

Serves 2

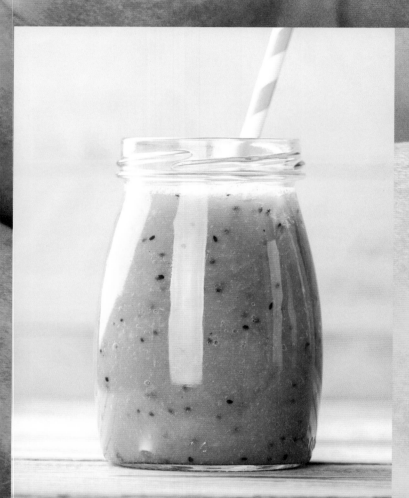

½ cup kale

2 cups fresh (or frozen) peaches, roughly chopped

¼ cup vanilla kefir or GoodBelly coconut water probiotic drink

1 tablespoon raw cashews

¼ teaspoon wheatgrass powder

1 tablespoon Mila chia seeds

½ teaspoon quandong powder

½ teaspoon Ahiflower oil

¼ cup filtered (or spring) water (optional)

Handful ice (optional)

KIWI PEAR SMOOTHIE

Serves 2

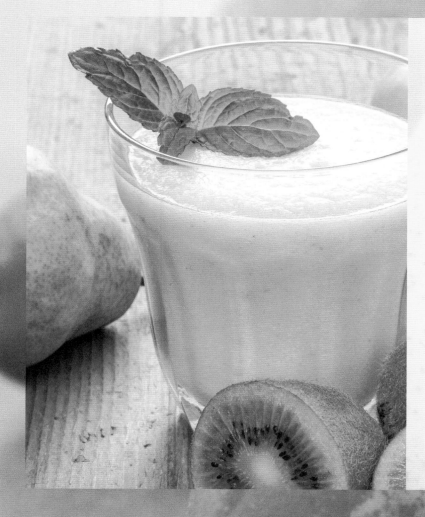

2 kiwifruits, sliced with skin on

1 large ripe pear

½ teaspoon kakadu plum powder

1 cup GoodBelly coconut probiotic drink

½ cup filtered (or spring) water

2 sprigs fresh spearmint or mint

1 cup fresh spinach

1 tablespoon Mila chia seeds

1 tablespoon raw hemp seeds

½ teaspoon Ahiflower oil

Handful ice (optional)

PINEAPPLE SPEARMINT SMOOTHIE

Serves 2

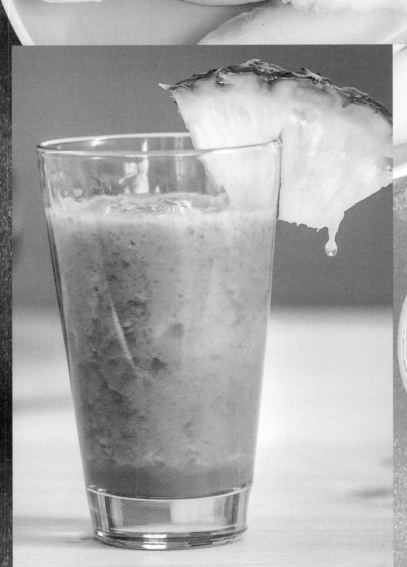

1½ cups pineapple, roughly chopped

2 fresh sprigs spearmint or mint

1 banana, peeled

1 tablespoon Mila chia seeds

1 teaspoon maca powder

¼ cup homemade (or unsweetened store-bought) almond milk

½ cup filtered (or spring) water or ½ cup cactus water (see Resources on where to buy)

½ teaspoon Ahiflower oil

Handful ice (optional)

ULTIMATE KIWI GREENS SMOOTHIE

Serves 2

4 kiwifruits, sliced with skin on

2 cups filtered (or spring) water

½ cup Harmless Harvest coconut water

½ lemon, slightly skinned (leave some peel on)

½ banana, peeled

1 apple (pink lady or fuji, or whatever is in season)

3 sprigs fresh mint

1 leaf chard

3 leaves sweet red lettuce or romaine

1 tablespoon raw hemp seeds

1 teaspoon spirulina/chlorella mix

1 teaspoon maca powder

1 tablespoon Mila chia seeds

½ teaspoon Ahiflower oil

Handful fresh parsley

Handful ice (optional)

WATERMELON CACTUS PEAR SMOOTHIE

Serves 2

2 cups watermelon, diced

1 cactus pear, peeled

1 banana, peeled

1½ teaspoons maqui powder

¼ teaspoon Himalayan (or Celtic) sea salt

½ cup GoodBelly coconut probiotic drink

½ cup filtered (or spring) water

1 teaspoon maca powder

1 tablespoon raw hemp seeds

1 cup raw fresh spinach leaves (optional)

1 teaspoon fresh lemon juice

½ teaspoon Ahiflower oil

Handful dried goji berries

Handful of ice (optional)

KAKADU PLUM SMOOTH

Serves 2

2 large red plums or pluots, diced with skin on

1 cup fresh (or frozen) strawberries

½ cup GoodBelly coconut probiotic drink
or plain coconut water

½ teaspoon kakadu plum powder

1½ tablespoons Mila chia seeds

½ cup fresh (or frozen) raspberries

½ cup filtered (or spring) water

½ teaspoon Ahiflower oil

Handful ice (optional)

SPINACH KIWI PEAR SMOOTHIE

Serves 2

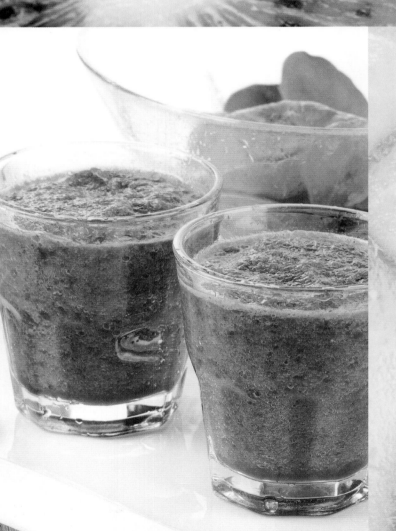

1 cup raw spinach

1 kiwifruit, peeled (optional)

1 bosc pear, roughly chopped with skin on

1 lemon, slightly skinned (leave some peel on)

1 tablespoon raw hemp seeds

½ teaspoon kakadu plum powder

1 tablespoon unhulled raw sesame seeds

3 fresh dates, soaked in water for ½ hour to soften

1 fresh (or frozen) banana, peeled

2 dried shiitake mushrooms

½ cup kefir yogurt or 1 tablespoon prebiotic powder
(see Resources on where to buy)

½ cup homemade almond milk or unsweetened
store bought (see Resources on where to buy)

1 cup filtered (or spring) water

½ teaspoon Ahiflower Oil

Handful of ice (optional)

COCONUT MATCHA LAVENDER SMOOTHIE

Serves 2

1 tablespoon raw shredded coconut

1½ teaspoons matcha powder

1 teaspoon dried lavender flowers
(see Resources on where to buy)

1 banana, peeled

1 tablespoon Mila chia seeds

1 tablespoon raw hemp seeds

3 Brazil nuts

1 cup homemade almond (or cashew) milk

½ cup GoodBelly coconut water probiotic drink

½ teaspoon vanilla extract (non-alcoholic if possible)

½ teaspoon Ahiflower oil

Handful ice (optional)

MATCHA PEACH SMOOTHIE

Serves 2

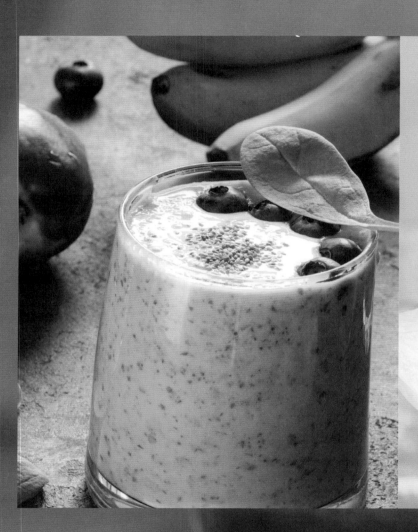

1½ teaspoons green matcha powder

2 ripe peaches, roughly chopped

½ cup low-fat kefir yogurt

½ cup GoodBelly coconut probiotic drink or Harmless Harvest coconut water

1½ teaspoons maca powder

½ teaspoon quandong powder

1 tablespoon raw hemp seeds

1½ cups fresh spinach leaves

2-inch cube organic sprouted tofu

1 banana, peeled

1 cup filtered (or spring) water

½ teaspoon Ahiflower oil

PAPAYA MAUI SMOOTHIE

Serves 2

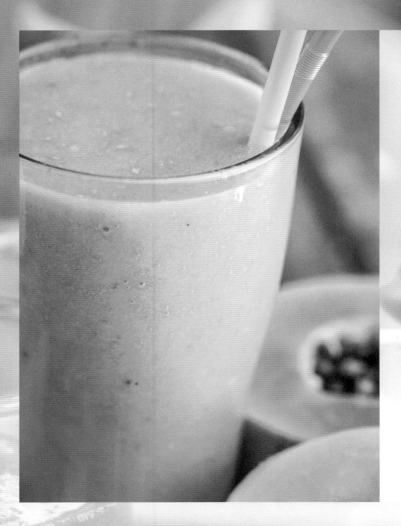

1 strawberry papaya, skin and seeds removed

1 apple banana (or regular banana), peeled

1½ cups GoodBelly coconut probiotic drink or Harmless Harvest coconut water

2 tablespoons raw hemp seeds

1 tablespoon Mila chia seeds

½ teaspoon wheatgrass

2 Brazil nuts

½ teaspoon Ahiflower oil

Handful ice (optional)

TASTY TROPICAL SAPOTE FRUIT SMOOTHIE

Serves 2

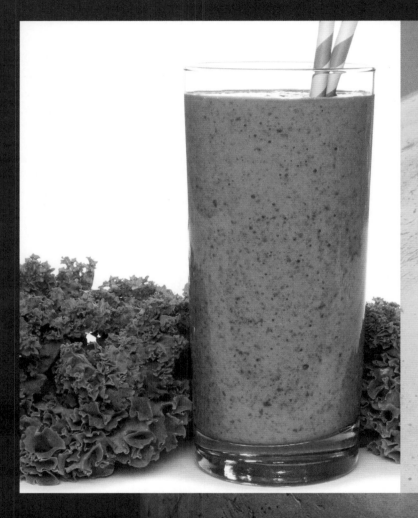

1 very soft green sapote, skin and seeds removed
(see Resources on where to buy)

1 cup kale

1 small apple banana (or regular banana)

2 tablespoons raw hemp seeds

2 cups GoodBelly coconut probiotic drink
or Harmless Harvest coconut water

3 Brazil nuts

1 tablespoon Mila chia seeds

¼ cup filtered (or spring) water

½ teaspoon Ahiflower oil

Handful ice (optional)

COZY WARM PEAR SMOOTHIE

Serves 2

2 cups poached pears with syrup*

2 tablespoons Mila chia seeds

3 tablespoons coconut kefir (see kefir recipe, page 107) or store-bought low-fat Greek yogurt

1 tablespoon raw hemp seeds (optional)

½ teaspoon Ahiflower oil

* In a saucepan, boil 3 pears (peeled and quartered) with 3 cups filtered or spring water for 30-40 minutes over a medium-high heat.

GUAVA STRAWBERRY SMOOTHIE

Serves 2

1–2 frozen guava puree packets (see Resources on where to buy) or 1 cup fresh guava, peeled

1 cup fresh (or frozen) strawberries

2 tablespoons coconut kefir (see kefir recipe, page 107) or store-bought low-fat Greek yogurt

1½ cups fresh coconut water or filtered/spring water

1 tablespoon Mila chia seeds

½ teaspoon riberry powder

Pinch stevia powder (optional)

½ teaspoon Ahiflower oil

AUSSIE LEMON BASIL SMOOTHIE

Serves 2

2 lemons, slightly skinned (leave some peel on)

2 sprigs fresh basil, leaves only

½ cup raw spinach

1 large apple, skin on

½ teaspoon kakadu plum powder

2 tablespoons Mila chia seeds

1 cup filtered (or spring) water

Handful raw cashews

½ teaspoon Ahiflower oil

Handful ice (optional)

CHICKPEA MISO BROTH

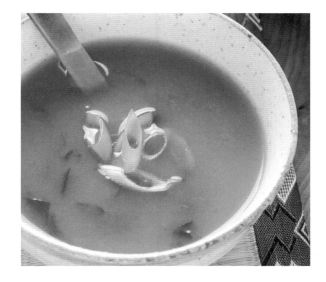

4 tablespoons chickpea miso paste

8 cups filtered (or spring) water

DIRECTIONS

1. Pour water into a steel pot and heat over a low heat.

2. Mix in chickpea miso paste and mash with a spoon until dissolved for 10 minutes. You're done – it's that easy!

3. Enjoy now, refrigerate for up to 1 week or freeze for several months.

ARTICHOKE LEMON SOUP BOWL

Serves 4

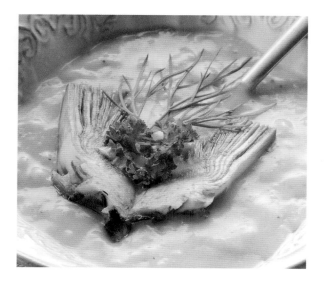

5 artichoke hearts, rinsed well

1 cup quinoa, rinsed

1½ cups cold water

3 cups raw spinach, chopped

1 tablespoon virgin olive oil

1½ yellow onions, chopped

2 large cloves garlic, minced

3 cups homemade Golden Mineral Broth (see recipe) or store-bought organic low-sodium broth

1½ teaspoons fresh thyme

1½ tablespoons fresh squeezed lemon juice, plus extra to serve

½ teaspoon Himalayan sea salt

½ teaspoon ground black pepper, plus extra to taste

½ cup raw cashews

1½ cups Italian flat leaf parsley chopped up

1½ tablespoons Ahiflower oil

4 tablespoons raw hemp seeds, to garnish

DIRECTIONS

1. Cut bottom stem off artichokes and trim top ends of all outer hard leaves. Place into a steamer with 4–5 inches of water. Cook for about 40 minutes, or until leaves pull off easily. Remove from stove and run under cold water.

2. Add quinoa to a 2-quart pot and add water. Bring to a boil and then reduce to medium-low and simmer for 10–12 minutes until fluffy. Remove from heat and let cool for 5 minutes. Add about ½ cup of quinoa to 4 soup bowls. Top quinoa in each bowl with ½ cup of the raw spinach.

3. Remove all leaves from the cooked artichoke and use a teaspoon to remove the furry part of choke. Slice artichoke heart up into small chunks and set aside until cool.

4. In a saucepan over medium heat, warm the olive oil. Add the onions and garlic and cook until translucent, about 5 minutes. Add Golden Mineral Broth, thyme, lemon juice, salt and pepper and bring to a simmer. Remove from the heat.

5. Pour soup into a high-speed blender with artichoke chunks, cashews, parsley and Ahiflower oil. Blend on soup mode until smooth, warm and creamy.

6. Ladle soup into soup bowls over spinach and quinoa. Top with raw hemp seeds and season with pepper to taste.

CURRIED BUTTERNUT SQUASH SOUP BOWL

Serves 4

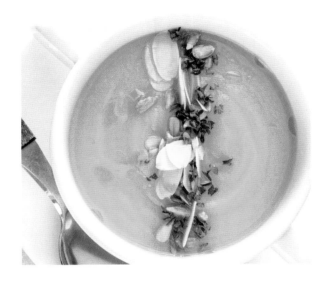

1½ tablespoons virgin olive oil

1 yellow onion, chopped

1 teaspoon yellow curry powder

½ cup Coconut Secret Aminos Garlic Sauce

1 clove garlic, minced

4 cups butternut squash, cut into 1-inch cubes

1½ cups Elaine's Essential Bone Broth (see recipe) or store-bought organic bone broth (if vegetarian, substitute with Golden Mineral Broth or store-bought organic low-sodium broth)

2 pinches Himalayan sea salt

2 pinches black pepper, plus extra to taste

1 cup quinoa, rinsed

1½ cups water

3 cups raw kale, chopped

1½ tablespoons Ahiflower oil

4 tablespoons raw hemp seeds, to garnish

DIRECTIONS

1. In a saucepan over medium heat, warm the olive oil. Add the onions and cook until translucent, about 5 minutes. Add the curry, Coconut Secrets and garlic and cook until fragrant, about 5 minutes. Add the squash, bone broth, salt and pepper, increase the heat to medium and simmer for 7 minutes. Reduce the heat to low and maintain a simmer. Cover and cook until the squash is tender when pierced with a fork, about 20 minutes. Remove from heat and leave to cool.

2. Add quinoa to a 2-quart pot and add water. Bring to a boil and then reduce heat to medium-low, simmering for 10–12 minutes until fluffy. Remove from heat and let cool for 5 minutes. Add about ½ cup of quinoa to 4 soup bowls. Top quinoa in each bowl with ½ cup of the raw spinach.

3. Pour soup into a high-speed blender with Ahiflower oil and blend on soup mode until smooth, hot and creamy.

4. Ladle soup into soup bowls over spinach and quinoa. Top with raw hemp seeds and season with pepper.

SAFFRON ASPARAGUS SOUP BOWL

Serves 4

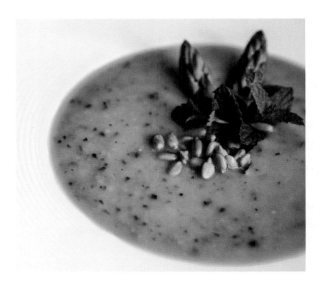

1½ tablespoons extra-virgin olive oil

1 yellow onion, chopped

2 stalks celery, leafy ends removed, chopped

1 packet or teaspoon saffron threads

1 clove garlic, minced

1 bunch fresh asparagus, chopped into 1-inch pieces

3 cups Elaine's Essential Bone Broth (see recipe) or store-bought organic bone broth (if vegetarian, substitute with Golden Mineral Broth or store-bought organic low-sodium broth)

Juice of ½ lemon

1 teaspoon chickpea miso

½ teaspoon Himalayan sea salt

½ teaspoon black pepper, plus extra to taste

1 cup quinoa

1½ cups water

3 cups raw spinach, chopped

1½ tablespoons Ahiflower oil

4 tablespoons sunflower seeds or almonds, crushed and warmed

DIRECTIONS

1. In a saucepan over medium heat, warm the olive oil. Add the onions and celery. Cook until translucent, about 5 minutes. Add the saffron and garlic and cook until fragrant, about 5 minutes. Add the asparagus, bone broth, lemon, chickpea miso, salt and pepper, increase the heat to medium and simmer for 7 minutes. Reduce the heat to low, maintain a simmer for another 5 minutes. Remove from heat and leave to cool.

2. Add quinoa to a 2-quart pot and add water. Bring to a boil and then reduce heat to medium-low, simmering for 10–12 minutes until fluffy. Remove from heat and let cool for 5 minutes. Add about ½ cup of quinoa to 4 soup bowls. Top quinoa in each bowl with ½ cup of the raw spinach.

3. Pour soup into a high-speed blender with Ahiflower oil and blend on soup mode until smooth, hot and creamy.

4. Ladle soup into soup bowls over spinach and quinoa. Top with sunflower seeds or warmed crushed almonds and pepper to taste.

CARAMELIZED ONION CARROT SOUP BOWL WITH PESTO OIL

Serves 4

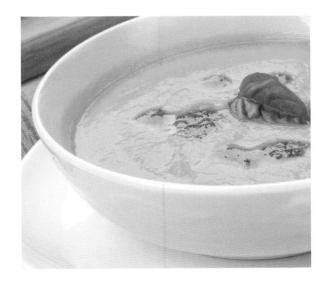

1½ tablespoons olive oil

2 large yellow onions, diced

1 stick celery, leafy ends removed, chopped

1½ pounds carrots, sliced into ¼-inch rounds

1 teaspoon fresh ginger, grated

Juice of 1 lemon

1 teaspoon apple cider vinegar

½ teaspoon black pepper, plus extra to taste

½ teaspoon Himalayan sea salt

2½ cups homemade Golden Mineral Broth (see recipe) or store-bought organic low-sodium broth

1 cup quinoa

1½ cups water

3 cups raw kale, chopped

1½ tablespoons Ahiflower oil

4 tablespoons almonds, crushed and warmed

Ahiflower Lemon Pesto Oil, to serve (see recipe)

DIRECTIONS

1. In a saucepan over low heat, warm the olive oil. Add the onions and saute for 45–50 minutes until onions are caramelized. Add celery, carrots and ginger, lemon, apple cider vinegar, pepper, salt and stir in with onions. Cook about 10 minutes. Add the Golden Mineral Broth and increase the heat to medium and simmer for ten minutes. Reduce the heat to low, maintain a simmer for five minutes more. Turn off and let cool.

2. Add quinoa to a 2-quart pot and add water. Bring to a boil and then reduce heat to medium-low, simmering for 10–12 minutes until fluffy. Remove from heat and let cool for 5 minutes. Add about ½ cup of quinoa to 4 soup bowls. Top quinoa in each bowl with ½ cup of the raw spinach.

3. Pour soup into a high-speed blender with Ahiflower oil and blend on soup mode until smooth, hot and creamy.

4. Ladle soup into soup bowls on top of spinach and quinoa. Top with almonds, season with pepper and drizzle over Ahiflower Lemon Pesto Oil.

ROASTED KABOCHA JAPANESE PUMPKIN SOUP BOWL

Serves 4

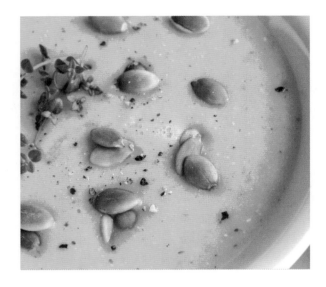

½ large kabocha pumpkin, seeded

2½ tablespoons extra-virgin olive oil

1 large yellow onion, diced

2 stalks celery, leafy ends removed, chopped

3 cloves garlic, minced

1¼ teaspoon ground cumin

½ teaspoon fresh ginger, grated

½ teaspoon ground coriander

½ teaspoon black pepper, plus extra to taste

½ teaspoon Himalayan sea salt

1 teaspoon apple cider vinegar

1½ cups Elaine's Essential Bone Broth (see recipe) or store-bought organic bone broth (if vegetarian, substitute with Golden Mineral Broth)

1 cup quinoa

1½ cups water

3 cups raw kale, chopped

1½ tablespoons Ahiflower oil

½ cup raw pumpkin seeds (not from kabocha pumpkin), warmed

½ cup raw sunflower sprouts

DIRECTIONS

1. Pre-heat oven to 375°F degrees. Put pumpkin on a baking tray and drizzle over ½ teaspoon of the olive oil. Roast for 30 minutes, or until the flesh is almost soft. Remove from oven and scoop out flesh.

2. In a saucepan over medium heat, warm remaining olive oil. Add onion and cook until translucent, about 5 minutes. Add pumpkin, celery, garlic, cumin, ginger, coriander, pepper, salt, apple cider vinegar and broth and cook until fragrant, about 10 minutes. Reduce to low, maintain a simmer, cover and cook until pumpkin is soft when pierced with a fork, about 10 minutes. Remove from heat and leave to cool.

3. Add quinoa to a 2-quart pot and add water. Bring to a boil and then reduce heat to medium-low, simmering for 10–12 minutes until fluffy. Remove from heat and let cool for 5 minutes. Add about ½ cup of quinoa to 4 soup bowls. Top quinoa in each bowl with ½ cup of the raw spinach.

4. Pour soup into a high-speed blender with Ahiflower oil and blend on soup mode until smooth, hot and creamy.

5. Ladle soup into soup bowls over spinach and quinoa. Top with pumpkin seeds, a handful of sunflower sprouts and pepper to taste.

ZUCCHINI CELERY SOUP

Serves 4

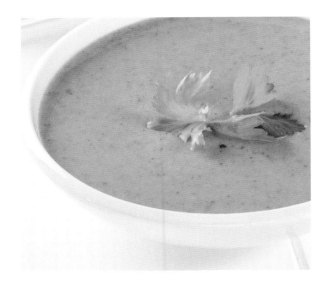

2 tablespoons extra-virgin olive oil

1 large yellow onion, diced

1 packet or teaspoon saffron threads

2 stalks celery, leafy ends removed, chopped

2 cloves garlic, minced

1½ teaspoons apple cider vinegar

3 small sprigs fresh thyme

1 teaspoon oregano

1 tablespoon raw hemp seeds

2½ small zucchinis, diced

3 cups Elaine's Essential Bone Broth (see recipe) or store-bought organic bone broth (if vegetarian, substitute with Golden Mineral Broth or store-bought organic low-sodium broth)

1 tablespoon chickpea miso paste

Juice of ½ lemon

½ teaspoon Himalayan sea salt

Black pepper

1 cup quinoa

1½ cups water

1½ tablespoons Ahiflower oil

2+ cups arugula, plus more if desired

½ cup almonds, crushed and lightly roasted

DIRECTIONS

1. In a saucepan over medium heat, warm the olive oil. Add the onions, saffron and celery. Cook until translucent, about 5 minutes. Add the garlic, apple cider vinegar, thyme, oregano, hemp seeds and cook until fragrant, about 5 minutes. Add the zucchini, broth, miso, lemon, salt and pepper, increase the heat to medium and simmer for 7 minutes. Reduce heat to low, maintaining a simmer for 5 minutes. Remove from heat and leave to cool.

2. Add quinoa to a 2-quart pot and add water. Bring to a boil and then reduce heat to medium-low, simmering for 10–12 minutes until fluffy. Remove from heat and let cool for 5 minutes. Add about ½ cup of quinoa to 4 soup bowls. Top quinoa in each bowl with around ½ cup of the arugula.

3. Pour soup into a high-speed blender with Ahiflower oil and blend on soup mode until smooth, hot and creamy.

4. Ladle soup into soup bowls on top of spinach and quinoa. Top with warmed crushed almonds and season with pepper.

GAZPACHO ROJO DE SEVILLA (COLD)SOUP BOWL WITH LEMON PESTO OIL

Serves 6

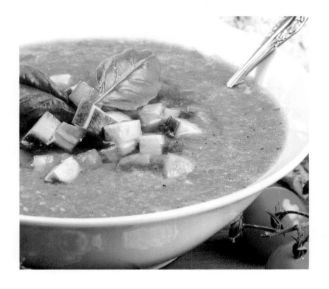

1½ tablespoons Ahiflower oil

2½–3 pounds ripe sweet tomatoes, skin on, stem and core removed, diced

1 large red or green bell pepper, stems and seeds removed, diced

1 large English cucumber, peeled and larger seeds removed

1 sweet Vidalia or Maui onion, diced

⅓ cup mirin cooking wine

1–2 tablespoons freshly squeezed lemon juice

2 teaspoons kakadu plum powder

2 tablespoons olive oil

½ teaspoon Himalayan sea salt

½ teaspoon black pepper ground, plus extra taste

1 cup of quinoa

1½ cups water

2+ cups arugula

Ahiflower Lemon Pesto Oil (see recipe)

DIRECTIONS

1. You will need to puree the soup in 2 batches. First, put Ahiflower oil, half the vegetables and half the mirin, lemon juice, plum powder, olive oil and salt and pepper in the blender. Blend on top speed for 20 seconds. Then repeat with the remaining ingredients and mix both batches together.

2. Chill for 1–2 hours or until cold.

3. Add quinoa to a 2-quart pot and add water. Bring to a boil and then reduce heat to medium-low, simmering for 10–12 minutes until fluffy. Remove from heat and let cool for 5 minutes. Add about ½ cup of quinoa to 4 soup bowls. Top quinoa in each bowl with around ½ cup of the arugula.

4. Ladle soup into soup bowls on top of arugula and quinoa. Top with Lemon Pesto Oil and season with pepper to taste.

PURSLANE (PORTULACA OLERACEA) CURRY SOUP BOWL

Serves 6

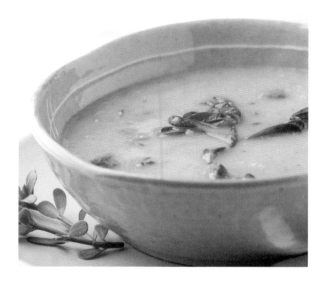

2 tablespoons olive oil

1 yellow onion, diced

2 tablespoons yellow curry powder

1 carrot, cut into ¼-inch rounds

2 cloves garlic, minced

2 tablespoons raw hemp seeds

2 tablespoons mirin cooking wine

8 cups purslane leaves, stems removed, plus extra to serve

2½-3 cups Chickpea Miso Broth (see recipe)

Juice of ½ lemon

1 teaspoon of Himalayan sea salt

Black pepper, plus extra to taste

1 baked or steamed russet potato, peeled and chopped

1 cup French black lentils, rinsed

1½ cups water

1 bay leaf

2+ cups raw spinach

1½ tablespoons Ahiflower oil

DIRECTIONS

1. In a saucepan over medium heat, warm the olive oil. Add the onions, curry powder and carrot. Cook until tender, about 5 minutes. Add the garlic, hemp seeds, potato, mirin and cook until fragrant, about 5 minutes. Add the purslane, broth, lemon, salt and pepper, increase the heat to medium and simmer for 7 minutes. Reduce the heat to low and maintain a simmer for 5 minutes. Remove from heat and leave to cool.

2. Add lentils to a 2-quart pot and add water and bay leaf. Bring to a boil and then reduce to medium-low to simmer for 25–30 minutes, until lentils are slightly tender. Remove from heat and let cool for 5 minutes. Drain. Add about ½ cup of lentils to 4 soup bowls. Top lentils in each bowl with around ½ cup of the spinach.

3. Pour soup into a high-speed blender with Ahiflower oil and blend on soup mode until smooth, hot and creamy.

4. Ladle soup into soup bowls on top of spinach and lentils. Top with chopped fresh purslane.

MARVELOUS MUSHROOM SOUP BOWL

Serves 4

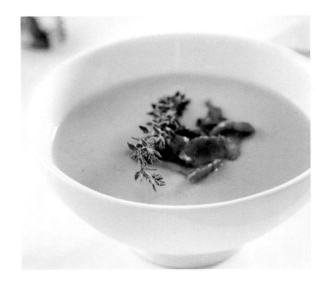

1½ tablespoons olive oil

½ yellow onion, chopped

1½ teaspoons fresh thyme, leaves only

1 clove garlic, minced

1¾ cup cremini mushrooms, chopped (leave ¾ cup for topping in each bowl before blending soup)

1 cup shiitake mushrooms, chopped

½ cup maitake mushrooms, chopped

5 cups Magic Mushroom Broth or (store-bought low sodium mushroom broth)

1 tablespoon raw hemp seeds

1 cup cauliflower florets, steamed and chopped

1 tablespoon mirin cooking wine

1 teaspoon freshly squeezed lemon juice

¼ teaspoon Himalayan sea salt

Pepper, plus extra to taste

3 cups raw spinach, chopped

1½ tablespoons Ahiflower oil

DIRECTIONS

1. In a saucepan over medium heat, warm the olive oil. Add the onions and thyme. Cook until tender, about 5 minutes. Add the garlic, half of each type of mushrooms, hemp seeds, cauliflower, mirin cooking wine and cook until fragrant, about 7 minutes. Add the broth, the remaining mushrooms, lemon, salt and pepper, increase the heat to medium and simmer for 7 minutes. Reduce to low and maintain a simmer for 5 minutes. Remove from heat and leave to cool.

2. Remove ¾ cup of mushrooms from the saucepan and set aside as a garnish.

3. Add ½ cup raw spinach to each soup bowl.

4. Pour soup into a high-speed blender with Ahiflower oil and blend on soup mode until smooth, hot and creamy.

5. Ladle soup into soup bowls on top of spinach. Top with the sauteed mushrooms and serve.

PEAR PEPPER SOUP BOWL

Serves 4

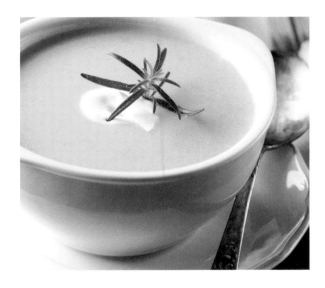

1 poblano pepper

2 tablespoons olive oil

1 yellow onion, chopped

2 large pears d'anjou or bartlett, peeled and diced

2 cloves garlic, minced

½ teaspoon ground cumin

1 tablespoon Italian flat leaf parsley, chopped

2 tablespoons raw hemp seeds

1½ cups Golden Vegetable Broth or Chickpea Miso Broth (see broth recipes) or store-bought organic low-sodium broth

¼ teaspoon Himalayan sea salt

Pepper

½ Anaheim or any green pepper with a kick, baked, skin removed and finely diced

1 large sweet yellow bell pepper, baked, skin removed and finely diced

1 cup quinoa

1½ cups water

2+ cups raw spinach

1½ tablespoons Ahiflower oil

DIRECTIONS

1. Bake poblano pepper at 425°F for 15 minutes, then broil for 8 minutes until the skin browns on top. When cool enough to handle, peel and quarter.

2. In a saucepan over medium heat, warm the olive oil. Add the onions, pears and garlic. Cook until translucent, about 7 minutes. Add the ground cumin, parsley, hemp seeds and baked peppers cook until fragrant, about 10 minutes. Add the broth, salt, pepper and diced peppers and simmer for 7 minutes. Remove from heat and leave to cool.

3. Add quinoa to a 2-quart pot and add water. Bring to a boil and then reduce heat to medium-low, simmering for 10–12 minutes until fluffy. Remove from heat and let cool for 5 minutes. Add about ½ cup of quinoa to 4 soup bowls. Top quinoa in each bowl with around ½ cup of the spinach.

4. Using a high-speed blender, add soup from saucepan and Ahiflower oil and blend on soup mode for only 10–15 seconds, leaving soup slightly chunky but hot and creamy.

5. Ladle soup into soup bowls on top of spinach and quinoa.

SWEET TOMATO BASIL LENTIL SOUP BOWL
Serves 4-6

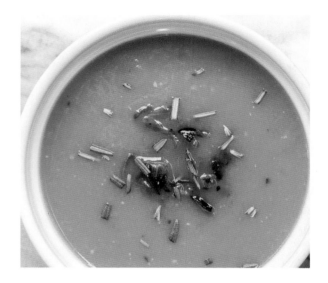

1 tablespoon olive oil

1 large sweet Vidalia onion, diced

1 stalk celery, leafy ends removed, chopped

1½ cloves garlic, minced

½ cup raw cashews

3 medium heirloom tomatoes or 8 small plum tomatoes

1 can organic (BPA-free) stewed tomatoes or 2 extra tomatoes

1 teaspoon maple syrup or coconut crystals

¼ cup dried goji berries

2 cups Golden Vegetable Broth (see recipe)
or store-bought low-sodium vegetable broth

¼ cup fresh basil, minced

¼ teaspoon Himalayan sea salt

Black pepper, plus extra to taste

1 cup French black lentils, rinsed

1½ cups water

2+ cups raw kale

1½ tablespoons Ahiflower oil

½ cup almonds, slightly roasted and crushed

DIRECTIONS

1. In a saucepan over medium heat, warm the olive oil. Add the onions, celery and garlic. Cook until translucent, about 7 minutes. Add the raw cashews, fresh and canned tomatoes, syrup and dried goji berries cook until fragrant, about 10 minutes more. Add the broth, basil, salt and pepper to taste and simmer for 7 minutes more. Remove from heat and leave to cool.

2. Add lentils to a 2-quart pot and add water and bay leaf. Bring to a boil and then reduce to medium-low to simmer for 25–30 minutes, until lentils are slightly tender. Remove from heat and let cool for 5 minutes. Drain. Add about ½ cup of lentils to 4 soup bowls. Top lentils in each bowl with around ½ cup of the kale.

3. Pour soup into a high-speed blender with Ahiflower oil and blend on soup mode until smooth, hot and creamy.

4. Ladle soup into soup bowls on top of kale and lentils.

MUSHROOM CHILI

Serves 6

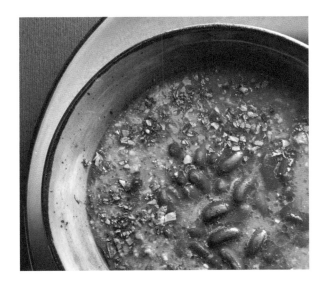

1 tablespoon olive oil

1 large sweet Vidalia onion, diced

2 large cloves garlic, minced

3 cups cremini mushrooms, chopped

½ teaspoon Himalayan sea salt

½ teaspoon black pepper

½ teaspoon ground cumin

1 teaspoon paprika

2½ tablespoons ground chili pepper

1 tablespoon fresh or dried oregano

2 tablespoons raw hemp seeds

1 cup maitake mushrooms, chopped

2 cups shiitake mushrooms, chopped

2 teaspoons superfood 10-mushroom blend (see Resources on where to buy)

1 cup sprouted extra-firm organic tofu, chopped

1 orange or yellow bell pepper, diced

1½ heaping teaspoons raw cacao powder

1½ cups Chickpea Miso Broth (see recipe in broth section)

2 cans or jars organic fire-roasted tomatoes (BPA free)

1 can kidney beans, drained and rinsed (BPA free)

3 teaspoons Ahiflower oil

Juice of 1 lime

1 cup quinoa

1½ cups water

3 cups fresh raw spinach, chopped

1 tablespoon almonds, lightly roasted, to garnish, or sliced scallions or grated parmesan

DIRECTIONS

1. In a saucepan over medium heat, warm the olive oil. Add the onions and garlic. Cook until translucent, about 7 minutes. Add the cremini mushrooms, salt, black pepper, ground cumin, paprika, chili pepper, oregano and hemp seeds. Cook until fragrant, about 10 minutes. Add the remaining mushrooms, mushroom blend, tofu, diced peppers, cacao powder, broth and simmer for 10 minutes. Then add in fire-roasted tomatoes and beans and cook on medium heat for 15 minutes. Remove from heat, add Ahiflower oil, lime juice, mix and cover.

2. Add quinoa to a 2-quart pot and add water. Bring to a boil and then reduce heat to medium-low, simmering for 10–12 minutes until fluffy. Remove from heat and let cool for 5 minutes. Add about ½ cup of quinoa to 4 soup bowls. Top quinoa in each bowl with around ½ cup of the spinach. Ladle chili on top of spinach and quinoa.

AHIFLOWER LEMON PESTO OIL

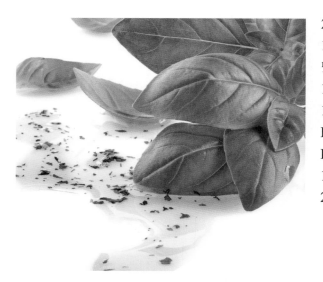

2 cups fresh basil, chopped

1 tablespoon freshly squeezed lemon juice

¼ cup Italian flat leaf parsley

1 clove garlic, minced

1 cup raw hemp seeds

Pinch of Himalayan sea salt

Pinch of black pepper

1 cup extra-virgin olive oil

2 tablespoons Ahiflower oil

DIRECTIONS

1. In a blender or small Cuisinart, add basil, lemon juice, parsley, garlic, hemp seeds, salt, pepper and oils.
2. Blend for a quick 30 seconds, pour into a bowl and leave to rest for 20 minutes at room temperature.
3. Drizzle 1 teaspoon of the oil over a soup of your choice.

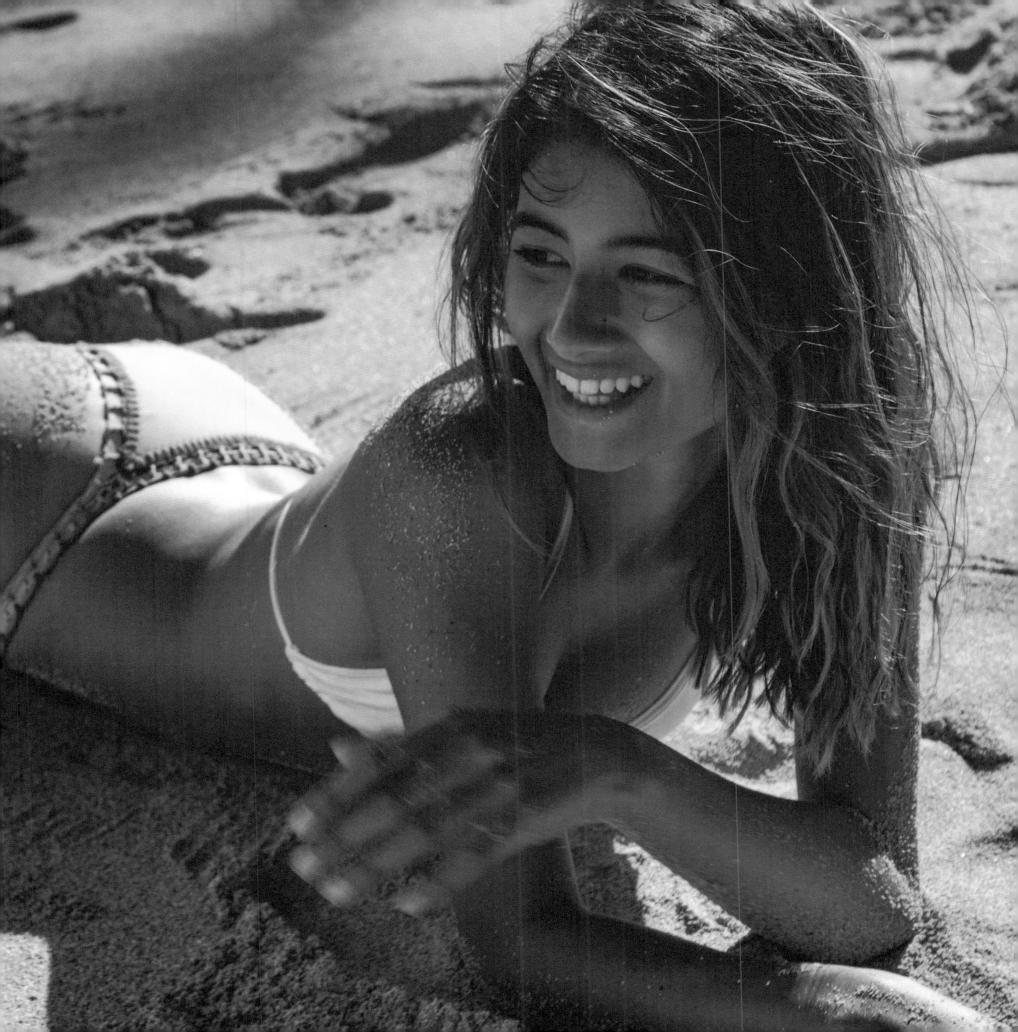

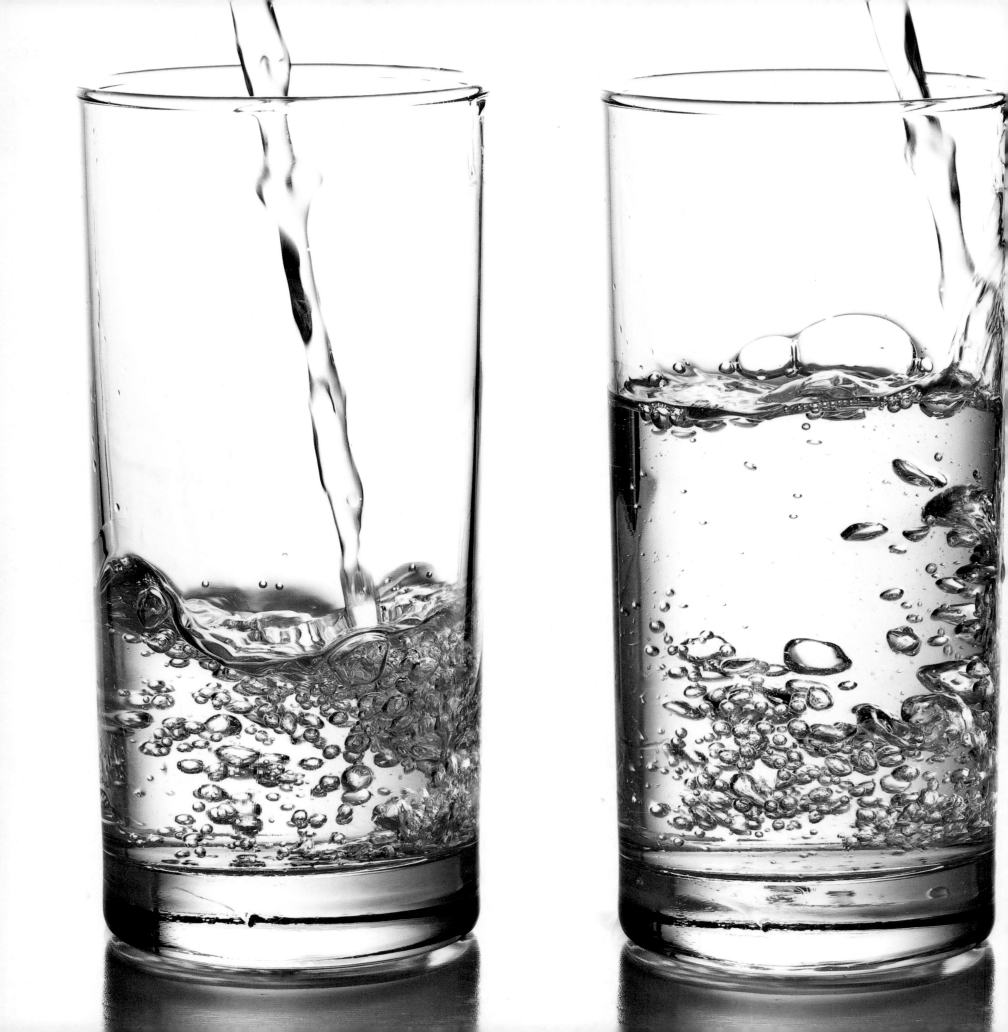

Chapter 10

WATER

We all know the benefits of keeping your body hydrated, but how important is it where your water comes from?

When we talk about sources of water, we usually think of tap water and bottled water. But there is a third option – my favorite – which is natural spring water. Natural spring water is one of the cleanest sources of water, and it tastes great. This type of water flows to the surface from a clean underground water source, be it a natural or mountain spring or an artesian well. When collected properly, the water is sparkling clean and free of most pollutants typically found in drinking water today.

Spring water (as well as glacial melt water) contains a good balance of minerals that are beneficial for our health. Mineral-rich water will usually have a neutral or slightly alkaline pH and is the healthiest water to drink. So, the more often we can drink alkaline water, the more it helps to neutralize our overall body acidity, helps to keep our bones and teeth strong and reduce the amount of free radical damage done to our bodies on a consistent basis.

Since water is one of the most critical components of the body, even minimal dehydration can hinder your sports performance and your ability to recover from any type of exercise. The reason for this is that your muscles are made up predominantly of water. Water composes 75 percent of muscle tissue and about 10 percent of fatty tissue. More importantly, water regulates your body temperature, aids digestion, protects vital organs, cushions joints, facilitates cellular communication, transports nutrients to the cells, and removes waste, including lactic acid, which is the main cause of exercise-related muscle soreness.[26]

THE MAGICAL HEALTH BENEFITS OF LEMON WATER

Lemons are a great source of vitamin C, magnesium, phosphorous, potassium, calcium, copper and bioflavonoids and have several medicinal properties. Do not throw away the skin, as it is also a very rich source of nutrients and can be used in smoothies and soups.

A great way to start your day is by drinking warm lemon water 30 minutes to an hour before you eat breakfast. Lemon water has an alkalizing effect and it stimulates the liver, which helps flush toxins out of your body. It also kills the bad-breath-causing bacteria in your mouth. Drinking water in the morning helps your gut by stimulating the production of hydrochloric acid, a very important ingredient needed in the stomach for digestion and waste elimination.[27]

Drinking lemon water regularly helps relieve indigestion, and bloating, and helps eliminate waste in the bowels more efficiently, easing constipation.[28]

HOW LEMON WATER CAN IMPROVE YOUR HEALTH

- Helps to purify and detoxify the blood, balance blood sugar levels, balance pH levels, and kill free radicals.
- The antioxidants in lemon water help fight damage to the skin caused by free radicals.
- Helps the body produce collagen, which keeps our skin looking young, fresh, smooth and supple.
- Boosts energy and mood in the morning without the caffeine rush.
- Helps nourish brain and blood cells due to its potassium content.
- Helps dissolve phlegm because of the citric acid present in lemon.
- Helps improve the immune system.

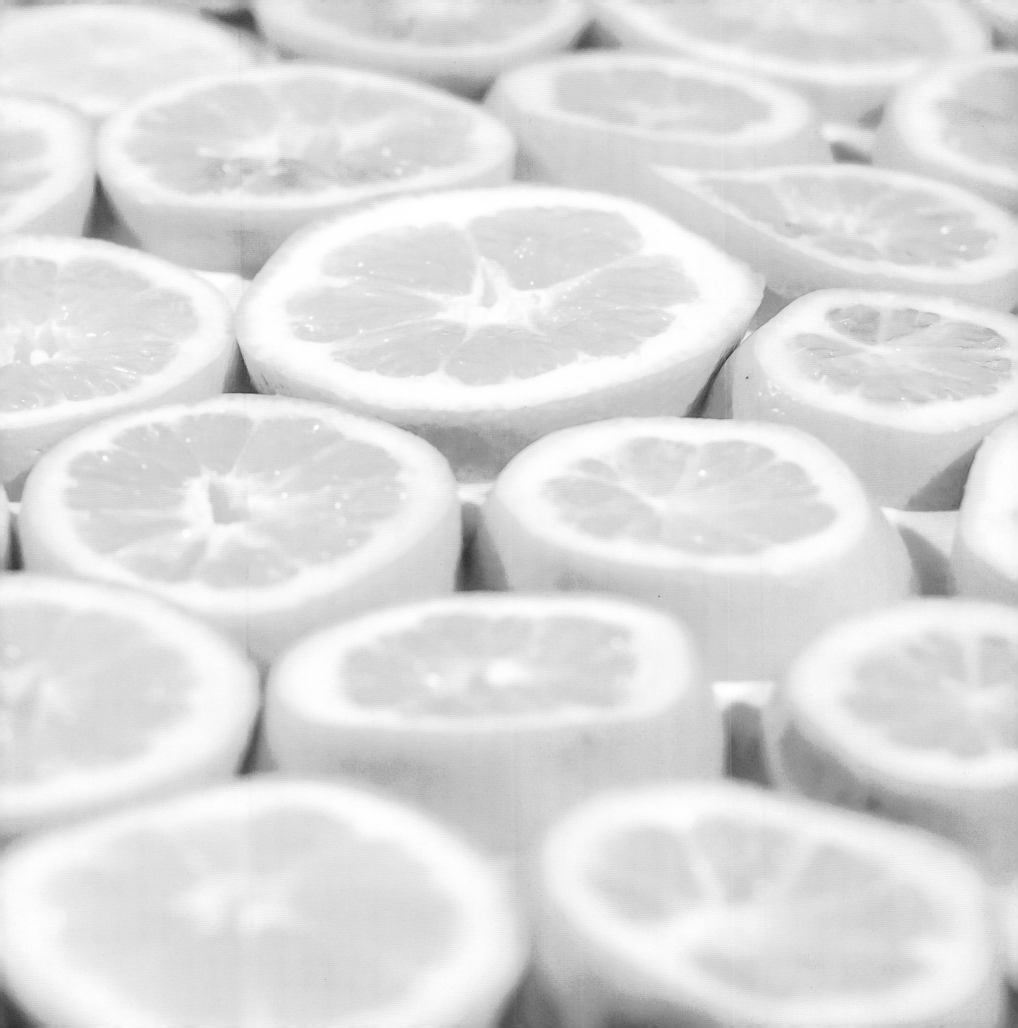

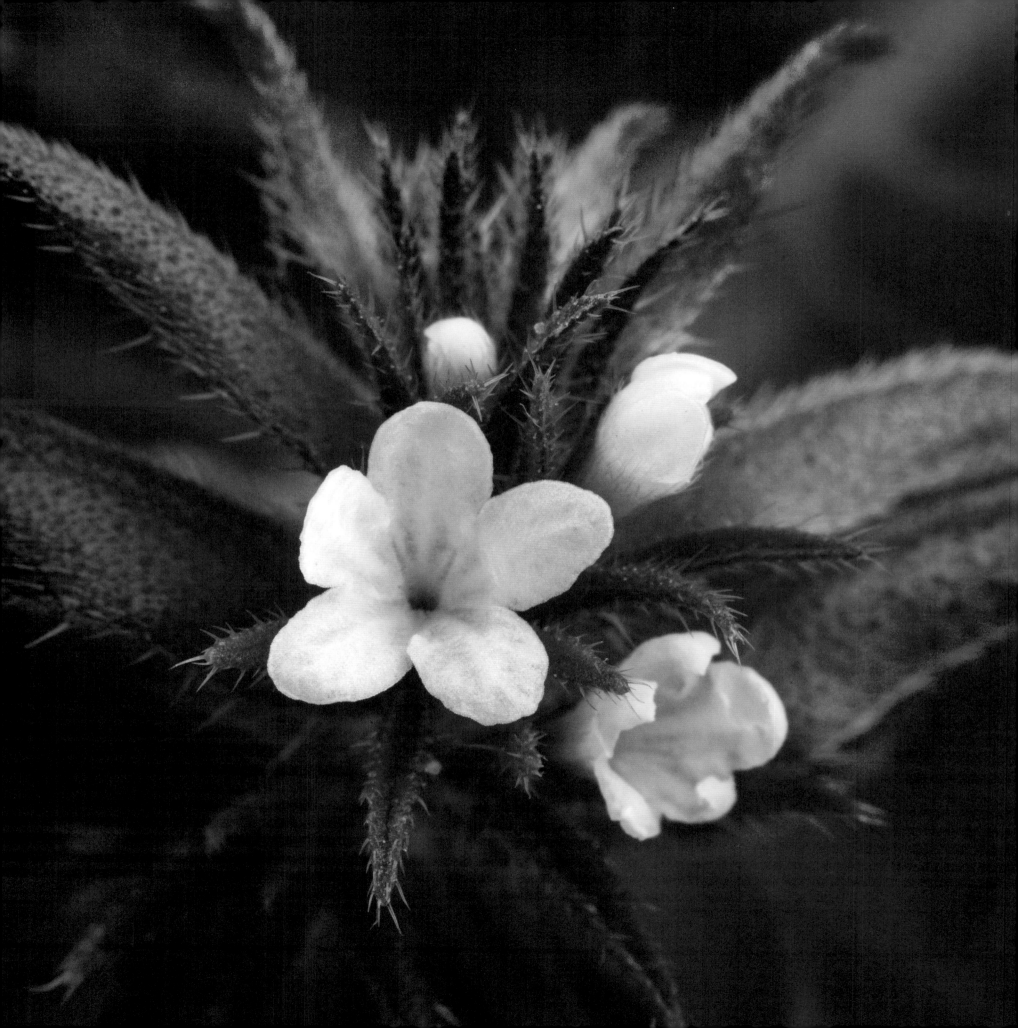

Chapter 11

OMEGA-3 FATTY ACIDS

Omega-3 fatty acids are polyunsaturated fatty acids (PUFAs) that are critical for brain, heart, joint and skin health. They are called "essential" fatty acids because our bodies cannot make them. They have to be obtained by eating foods rich in omega-3s, such as sardines, mackerel and salmon. Unfortunately, fish sources of omega-3s today are no longer safe because our oceans are polluted and many of our fish are filled with toxins, PCBs, heavy metals and mercury. Humans have also over-fished many wild fish species to the point that other marine life that rely on them, such as sea lions and pelicans, are starving.

AHIFLOWER OIL

Plant-based sources of omega-3s are a good alternative to fish-based sources. One of my favorite sources of omega-3s is Ahiflower oil, which contains the highest levels of stearidonic acid (SDA) and GLA (gamma-linolenic acid), both omega-3s that are commonly found in evening primrose and borage oils. Ahiflower oil has the richest and most balanced omega fatty acids 3, 6 and 9 from a single non-GMO plant. In addition to Ahiflower oil's more advanced plant-based omega-3 and omega-6 fatty acid benefits, Ahiflower oil now has recognized anti-inflammatory benefits. A recently published human clinical trial in the journal, *Nutrients*, showed that Ahiflower oil supports the body's natural anti-inflammatory and immune-modulation response.[29] This is especially useful for post-workout muscle and joint recovery, as well as for upper respiratory immune support.

ALGAL OIL

Another plant-based source of omega-3s is algal oil. Many consumers find the sensory (aroma and taste) experience of algal oils a little off-putting, but this is naturally part of the fact that they are very high in omega-3 lipids. Algal oils are derived from various specialized strains of algae grown in either ponds or closed loop vat systems. They are now commonly used in baby formula and in a variety of fortified beverages and dietary supplements. Algal oils are a valued non-marine fatty acid source; however, the cost of manufacturing them in a biotech environment also makes them more expensive than omega-rich oils such as Ahiflower oil.

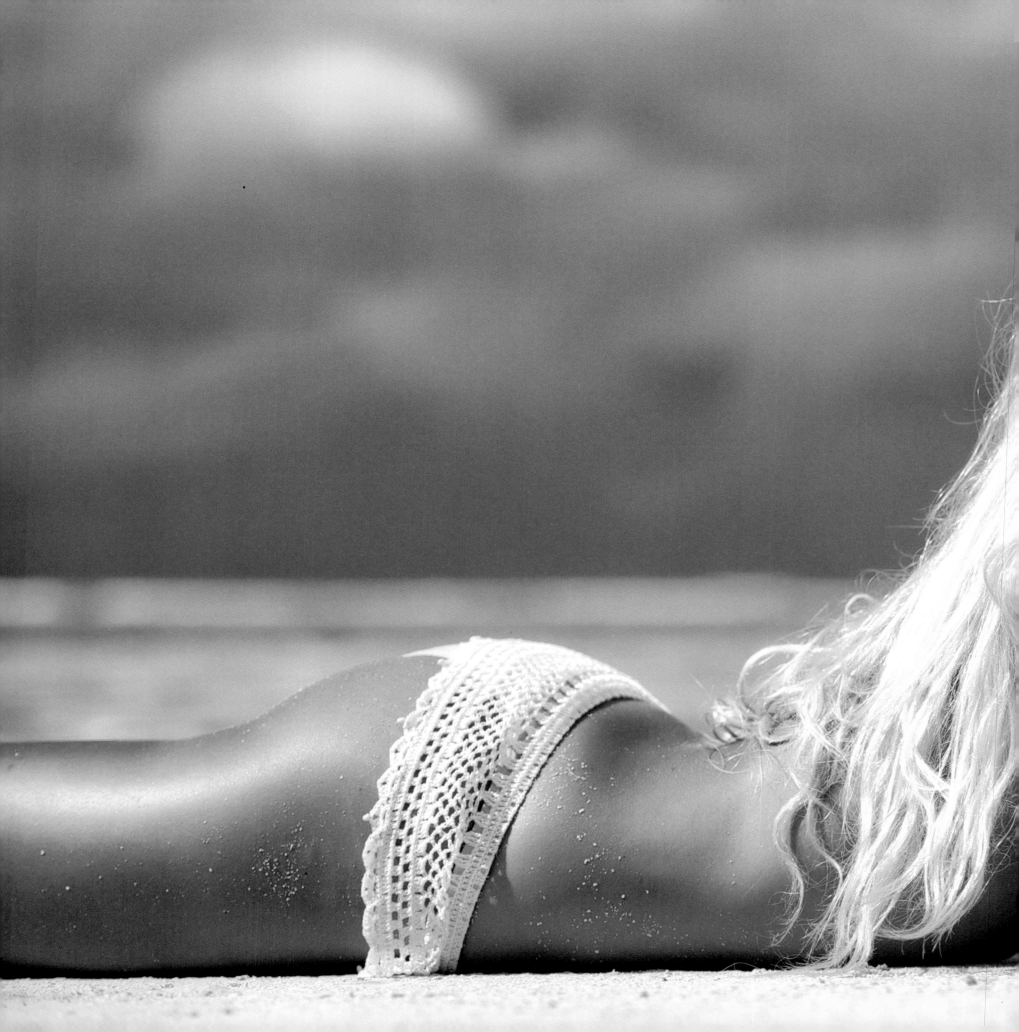

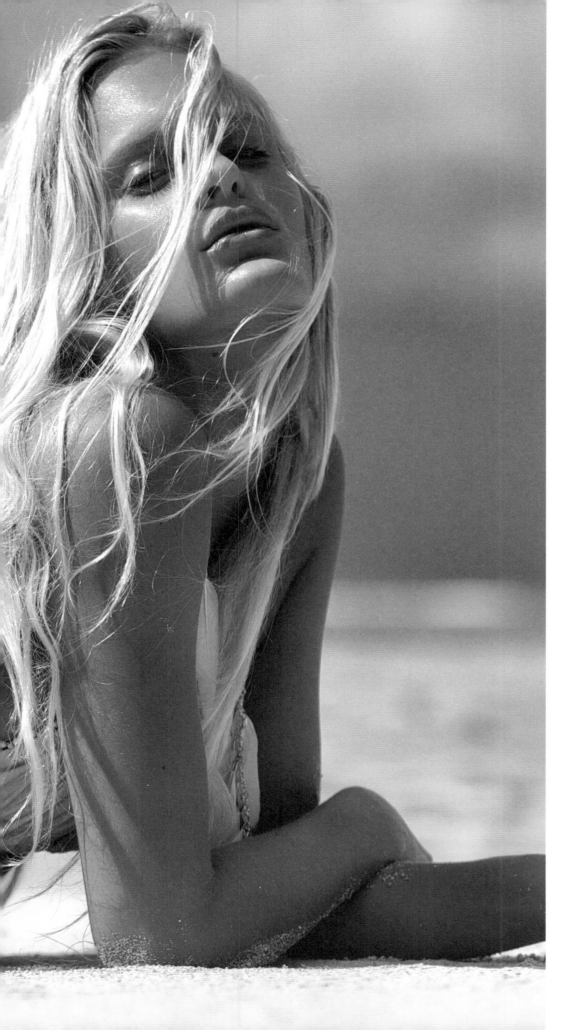

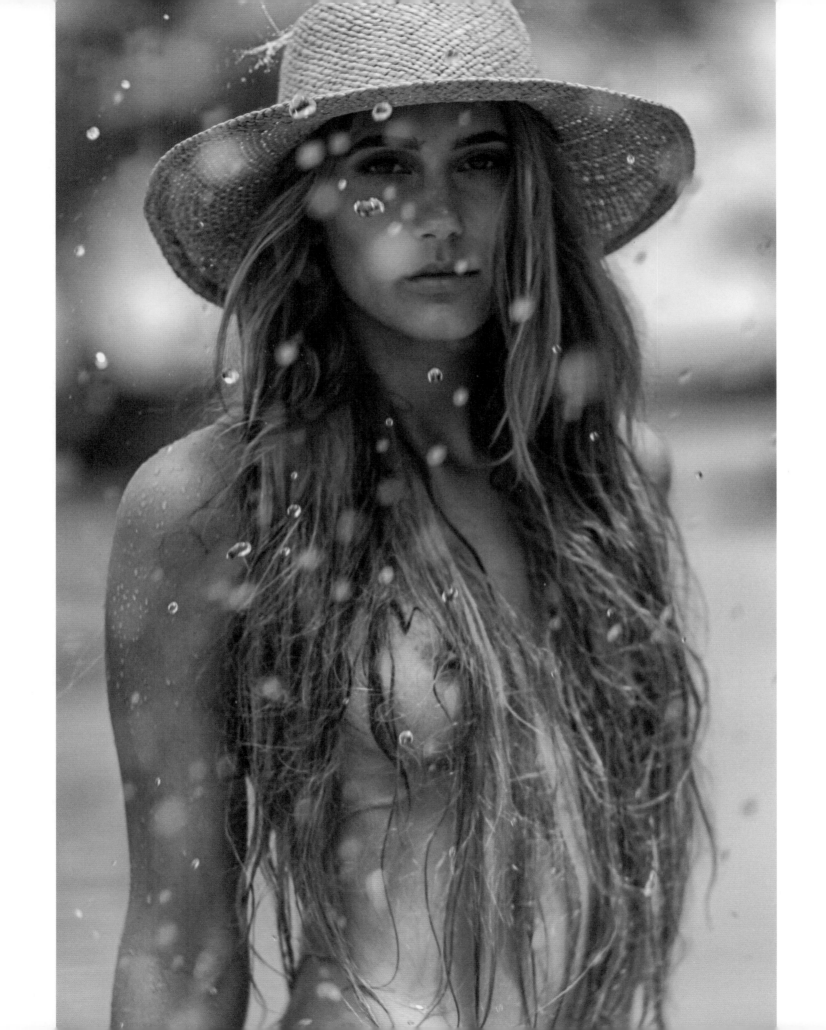

Chapter 12

THE SCIENCE BEHIND GLOWING SKIN & HAIR

Your skin and hair are an outward reflection of what is going on inside your body, so if you are wondering how to make your skin glow and your hair shine, you'll want to first assess what you're eating. In fact, what you eat is as important as the oils, serums and shampoos you use.

To cut to the chase, according to Dr. Lisa Miller, a naturopathic doctor in the San Francisco Bay area, the key to healthy skin and hair is to go heavy on greens, healthy fats and vitamin-rich foods, and light on salty and sugary items.[30]

The best way to reduce free radical damage and improve your skin and hair is through a healthy diet and lifestyle, rather than taking supplements. Antioxidant supplements can sometimes cause unwanted effects and are not as beneficial as eating whole plant foods. According to New York City nutritionist, Keri Glassman, eating foods filled with healthy fats – such as avocados, chia seeds, flax seeds, walnuts, bone broth, vegetable mineral broth and Ahiflower oil – helps reverse the breakdown of collagen, a skin-firming protein.[31] In addition, loading up on antioxidant-rich foods such as kakadu plums, kiwis and oranges helps slow down the effects of free radicals (unstable molecules that pillage through the body, destroying healthy cells and tissues) and protect your body from disease and signs of early aging. The vitamin A in cantaloupe, butternut squash, carrots and sweet potatoes helps reduce inflammation and promote cell turnover, which in turn helps combat acne. Other antioxidant sources include plant foods such as fruits or veggies, green or white teas, raw cocao, red wine, spices and herbs. My nutrient-dense superfood smoothies and soups will make visible improvements to your skin and hair in two weeks.

Cruciferous vegetables, such as broccoli, brussels sprouts, cabbage, cauliflower and kale contain a phytonutrient called sulforaphane that can help restore hormonal imbalances and help eliminate acne.[32]

IS YOUR HAIR THINNING OR FALLING OUT?

I have read countless articles about people who only drink juice and don't eat real food every day, and as a result, their hair starts falling out. This is because their diet is low in protein, which our body needs to work properly and produce energy. Protein does not have to be all animal protein; plant-based sources of protein such as lentils work just fine. The average person needs at least 20 grams of protein three times a day – more if they are an athlete. A 20-gram serving of protein is equivalent to three large eggs or five egg whites, a cup of tuna or two cups of chickpeas. Protein is not just about quantity, it's also about quality. If you don't eat animal foods, then it is a bit more challenging to get all the protein and essential amino acids that your body needs.

An easy way to make sure you're eating enough protein is to include a decent protein source in every meal or snack. Add nuts or beans to your salad, protein powder or almond butter to your smoothie or fruit snack, and beans or meat to your pasta.

Plant-based proteins that you can eat throughout the day include seeds such as hemp and sesame seeds/tahini (ground up is better because most people do not chew their food enough), and lentils or nuts, such as almonds or walnuts, which are not inflammatory.

VITAMINS FOR HEALTHY SKIN AND HAIR

Growing up, you were probably told that vitamin C would ward off all types of colds and other body ailments. That is true, but it is now known that vitamin C also plays a vital role in maintaining the health of your skin. Vitamin C is the key to the production of collagen, a protein that aids in the growth of cells and blood vessels and gives skin its firmness and strength.[33] It helps form scar tissue, prompts the skin to repair itself, and slows the rate of free radical damage. Free radicals are unstable molecules that damage collagen and cause wrinkles, dry skin and fine lines.[34]

Other vitamins that promote healthy skin include vitamins A, E, selenium and zinc. You also needs minerals, antioxidants, polyphenols, bioflavonoids, and omega-3 fatty acids. I recommend sourcing omega-3s from powerful, plant-based Ahiflower oil. Since our oceans are depleted and polluted, I do not recommend fish oils as a safe source of fatty acids.

Healthy, glowing skin requires healthy blood vessels. To have healthy blood vessels, you need to eat an array of brightly colored fruits and vegetables, which reduce inflammation and plaque formation, leading to better blood flow. Here is a suggested grocery list of items included in many of our smoothies and soups that will brighten your hair and complexion from the inside out:

Ahiflower oil, walnuts, hemp seeds, avocado, cucumber, mushrooms, pumpkin, lemon, sweet potato, yam, pomegranate, acorn squash, turmeric, fermented foods and greens, escarole, celery, watermelon, greens, beets, grapes, asparagus, coconut, kefir, kakadu plum, green tea, matcha, raw cacao, cinnamon, blueberries and asparagus.

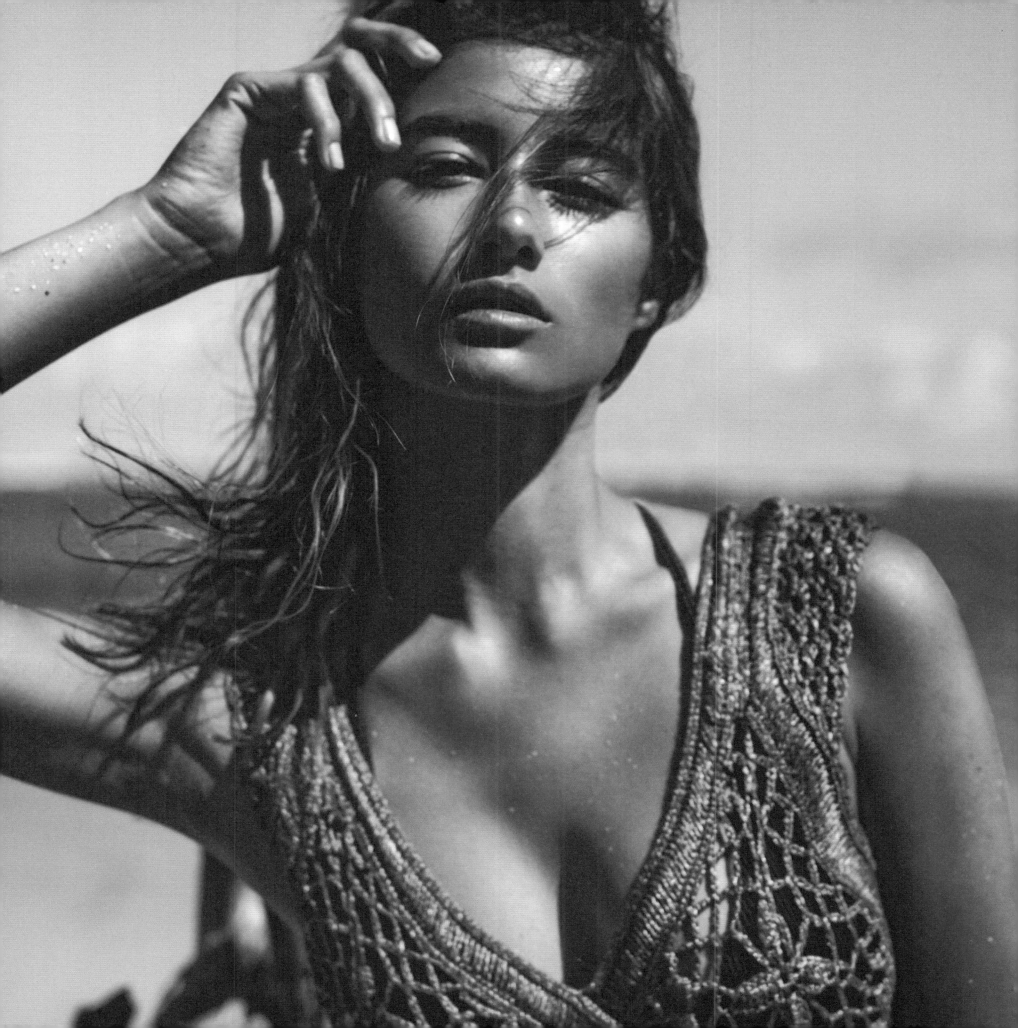

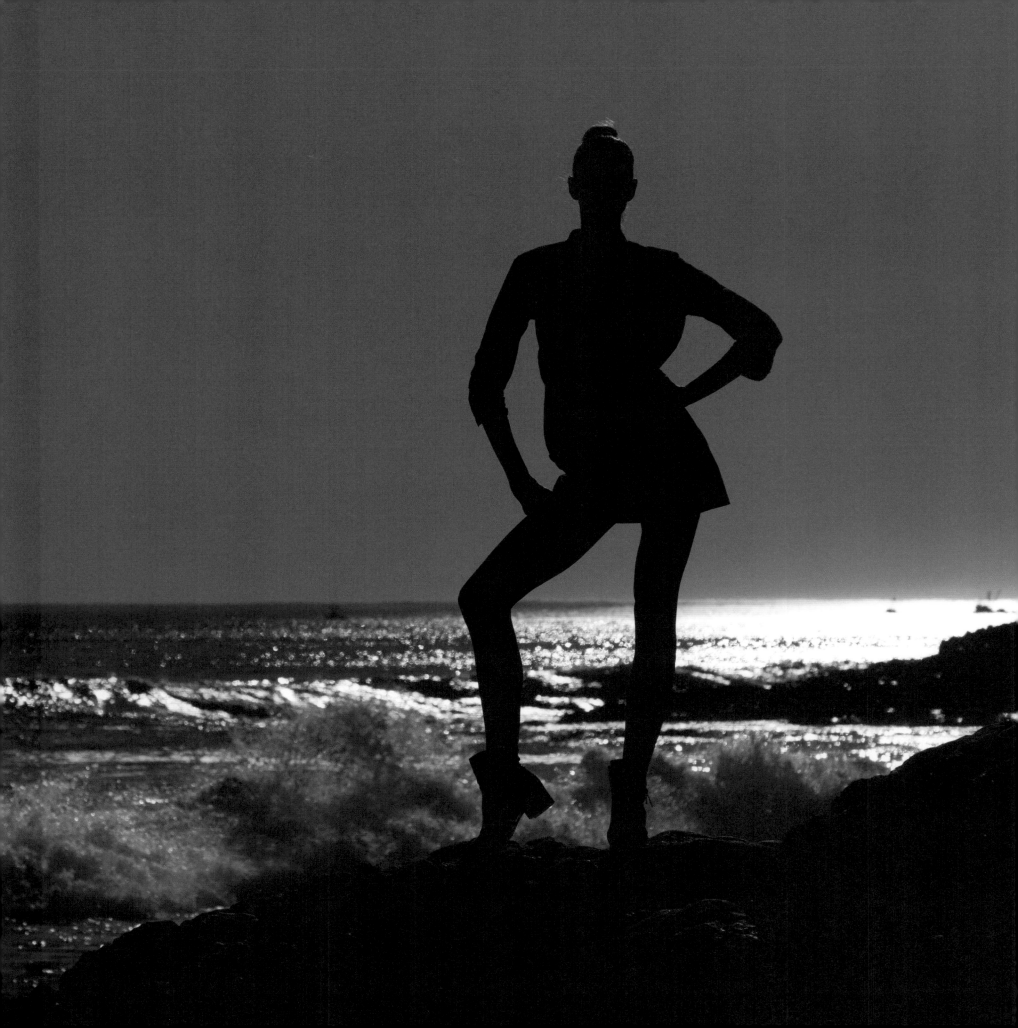

Chapter 13

KEEPING IT CLEAN

What goes on your skin goes into your bloodstream.

What you put on your skin and hair goes into your body, so ingredients really do matter. That's why I recommend a "clean" skin care practice. But what does that mean? Understanding the true nature of aging skin inside and out and addressing the causes at the cellular level, where change is possible, is mandatory for healthy skin and hair. What we eat must be clean, and the water we drink must be clean. Ultimately, the environment we live in must be clean.

I have reviewed and tried many skin care lines, and I am always on the hunt for the most natural lines. Some of my favorite clean, anti-aging skin care products include:

True Botanicals. Meticulously developed by thyroid cancer and melanoma survivor, Hillary Peterson, True Botanicals offers an entire skin care line that is organic and toxin-free. The Renew Collection is one of my favorites, as well as the nourishing shampoo. For skin care, I like the Renew Pure Radiance Oil, the Renew Cellular Repair Serum and the Vitamin C Booster.

DERMAdoctor. I like the Kakadu C 20% Vitamin C Serum with Ferulic Acid & Vitamin E. When you combine the vitamin C with these two antioxidants, it helps boost the vitamin C's power eightfold.

Marie Veronique. From this skin care brand, I love the Rejuvenating Night Oil, Extra Healing and Gentle Retinol Night Serum – both work wonders on my skin.

Biologique Recherche. All serums are beneficially potent and I really love their Crème Mask Vernix, which makes my face look and feel like a new baby's bum! The French evidently know skin care, as the entire line works extremely well.

Kat Burki. Their Rose Hip Revitalizing Serum has a trademarked "KB5 Complex", which works flawlessly with their purified, cold-pressed Rose Hip seed oil and their own stable form of vitamin C (that they call STAY C). This supports the skin's defenses and collagen integrity.

Goop by Juice Beauty & Gwyneth Paltrow. The Hollywood star's beauty line is all about transforming the chemistry of beauty safely. All products are formulated without the nasties (aka parabens, petroleum, pesticides, propylene or butylene glycols, phthalates, sulfates, PEGs, TEA, DEA, GMO, silicones, gluten, artificial dyes and synthetic fragrances). I incorporate the Enriching Face Oil into my daily routine. It's a potent oil that hydrates and leaves my skin super supple and soft. The Luminous Melting Cleanser is one of my favorites, as it completely removes any sign of dirt.

Tata Harper. We all need to use a purifying mask treatment at least once a week, and Tata Harper's Purifying Mask contains intense cleansing ingredients. The Reparative Moisturizer is a rich, ultra-hydrating face cream that is great for dehydrated skin in drier climates. Bonus: this entire skin care line smells wonderful.

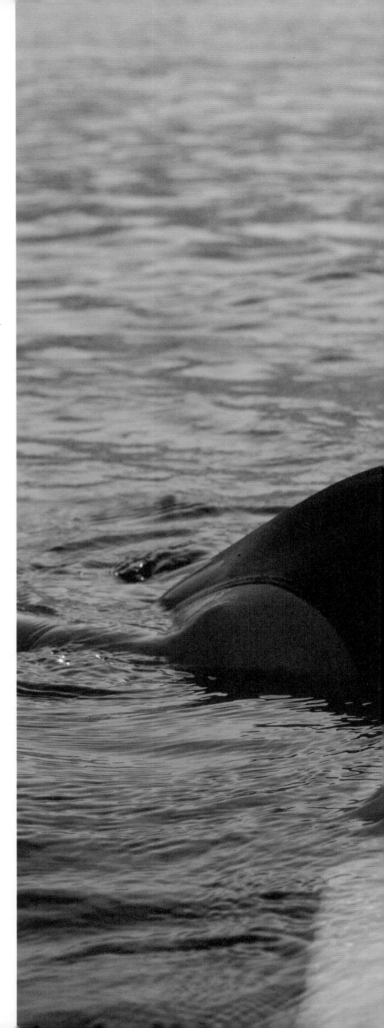

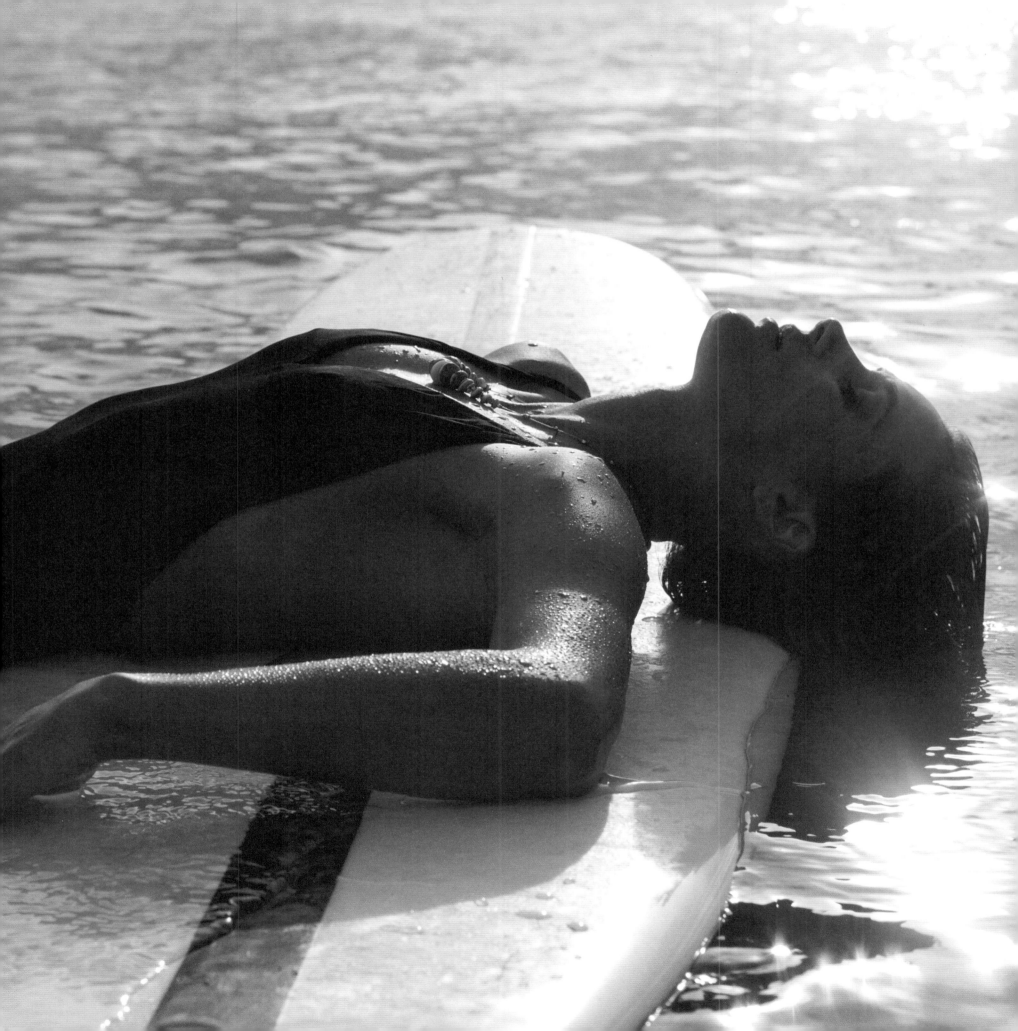

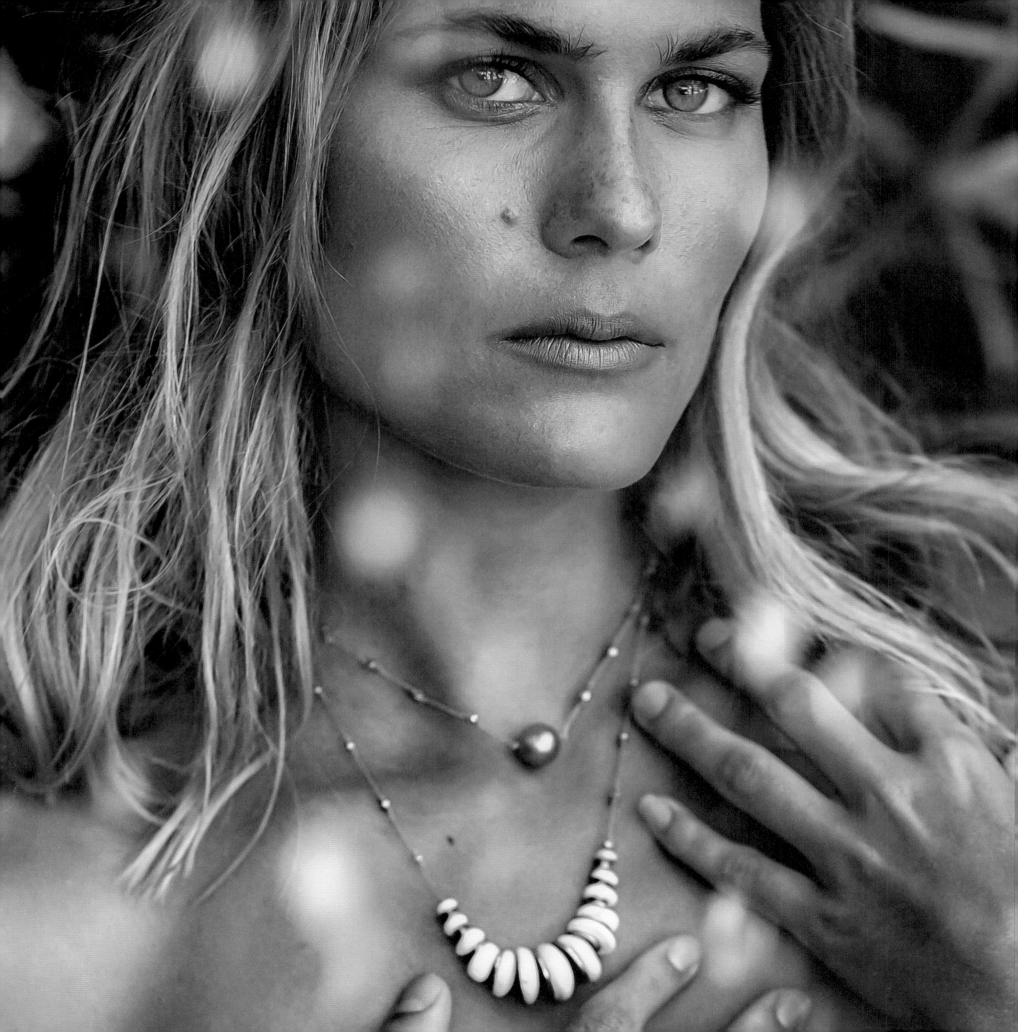

Chapter 14

SKIN TYPES AND ANTI-AGING ROUTINES

Finding the right skin care routine is much like finding that perfect pair of jeans. How many pairs have you tried on? Which work well on your body type? Low rise, high-rise, boot cut or straight? Do you like jeans with big pockets, small pockets or no pockets at all?

Your skin, like your body, changes throughout your life, so just as your jean style preference may evolve over time, so will your skin care routine. My advice is to book an appointment with an experienced, licensed skin care professional who can give you a personal skin analysis and determine what regime is best for you.

Skin type is all about genetics and ethnicity. While your skin can change over time, an individual's skin type is most often determined by the amount of oil your follicles produce. Skin types include normal, dry, combination, oily and sensitive. The goal in skin care is to balance the levels of oil and water in the skin and protect the acid mantle, the outermost layer of skin.

Another thing to keep in mind when determining skin type is the Fitzpatrick Scale.[35] This is a numerical classification scheme used by skin care professionals as part of their analysis. The Fitzpatrick scale measures the skin's ability to tolerate sun. Lighter skin is more sensitive to sun exposure, and burns more quickly. Darker skin produces more melanin and can tolerate more sun exposure.

Let's determine your Fitzpatrick number:

FITZPATRICK SCALE

1. *Very fair:* light hair, light eyes, freckles, always burns
2. *Fair:* Light hair, light eyes, burns
3. *Moderately fair:* fair, light or dark hair, can burn but tans over time
4. *Olive:* medium color, more pigment, rarely burns, tans easily
5. *Dark:* not very sensitive, tans
6. *Black:* rarely sun sensitive, tans easily

By matching your skin type with your Fitzpatrick number, you will better understand what products, procedures and treatments will work best for you.

SKIN CARE ROUTINES FOR DIFFERENT SKIN TYPES

I have outlined skin care routines for different skin types (normal, dry, oily, combination and sensitive), but the bottom line is that what works for one person may not work for another. Stay open to experimenting. Your skin will have different needs at different times throughout your life, so mix it up. If you are dry, add a hydrator and/or a moisturizer. If there is a special time of the month where your hormones wreak havoc on your skin, change up your routine to meet your immediate needs. If you will be in the sun all day, remember to apply sunscreen every two to three hours and at least 30 minutes before you expect to be exposed.[36]

NORMAL SKIN

Normal skin usually has a good balance of oil and water. It is predominantly blemish-free and has "normal"-sized follicles (pores). Normal is when the follicles in the T-zone (forehead, nose, chin) tend to be a little larger than those on the rest of the face, but are relatively small in size. The goal for skin care here is maintenance and protection.

NORMAL SKIN CARE ROUTINE

Morning

1. Rinse or cleanse, depending on how much residual oil or products you still feel on your face.
2. Use a toner.
3. Optional: Apply an antioxidant serum. My favorite is a vitamin C serum, with or without vitamin E.
4. Apply moisturizer (one with a good water to oil balance).
5. Apply eye cream.
6. Apply sunscreen (broad spectrum UVA/UVB with at least SPF 30).

Evening

1. Remove make-up and sunscreen. Personally, I love miceller water and oil cleansers.
2. Perform a double cleanse. That means wash and rinse the skin twice.
3. Use a toner.
4. Optional: Apply nutrient-rich serum.
5. Apply moisturizer.
6. Apply eye cream.

Note: It's important to exfoliate a few times every week. You can do this by using a mechanical cleansing brush, a cleanser with polishing beads or an enzyme mask. You may also want to incorporate a retinol product into your routine.

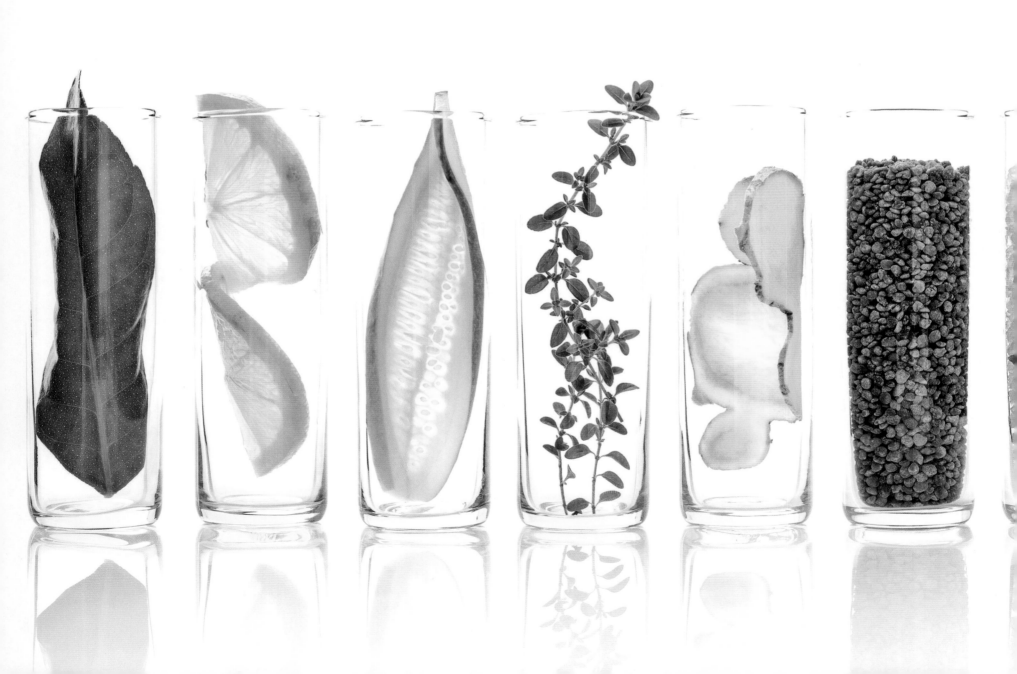

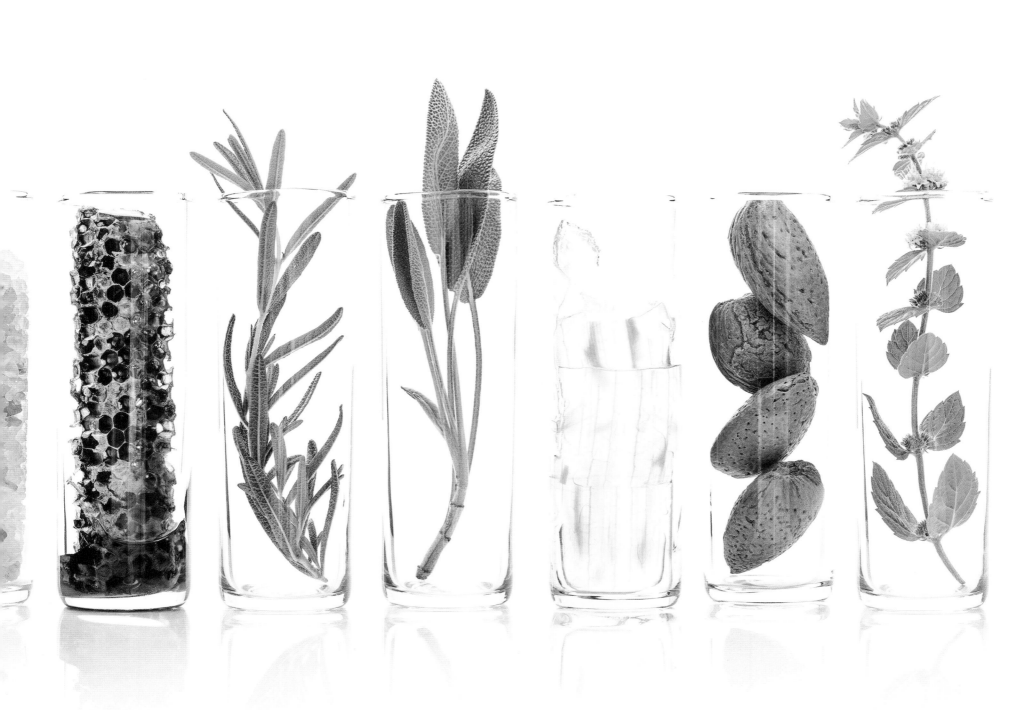

DRY SKIN

Dry skin is characterized by a lack of oil (alipidic) production. It usually occurs when pores are smaller. Skin is tight, possibly rough in texture and dry to the touch. Usually it is more sensitive because the acid mantle (outermost layer of skin) is compromised. This condition requires products that will help to maintain water levels and moisture in the skin. The goal is to hydrate and nourish the skin.

DRY VERSUS DEHYDRATED SKIN

Dry skin is when there is a lack of oil in the skin, whereas dehydrated skin is lacking water. All skin types can be dehydrated, even oily skin. Dehydrated skin can look and feel thinner. It can be flaky, tight and dry. This condition requires more hydration and moisture. Depending on your overall skin type one may need to use humectants and moisturizers to maintain skin balance.

DRY/DEHYDRATED SKIN CARE ROUTINE

Morning

1. Rinse or cleanse, depending on how much residual oil or products you still feel on your face.
2. Use a toner (calming or restorative).
3. Optional: Apply an antioxidant serum, preferably a vitamin C serum, with or without vitamin E.
4. Apply hydrating moisturizer.
5. Apply eye cream.
6. Apply sunscreen (broad spectrum UVA/UVB with at least SPF 30).

Evening

1. Remove make-up and sunscreen (try miceller water and oil cleansers).
2. Perform a double cleanse. That means wash and rinse the skin twice.
3. Use a toner to reset pH balance.
4. Optional: Apply a nutrient-rich serum.
5. Apply hydrating moisturizer (you may also use both a hydrator and a moisturizer separately).
6. Apply eye cream.

Note: For dry skin, exfoliate by using products containing enzymes or alpha-hydroxy acid. Physical forms of exfoliation can create more damage. Gentle is the name of the game! Try using a moisturizing mask a couple of times a week for deeper levels of moisture retention.

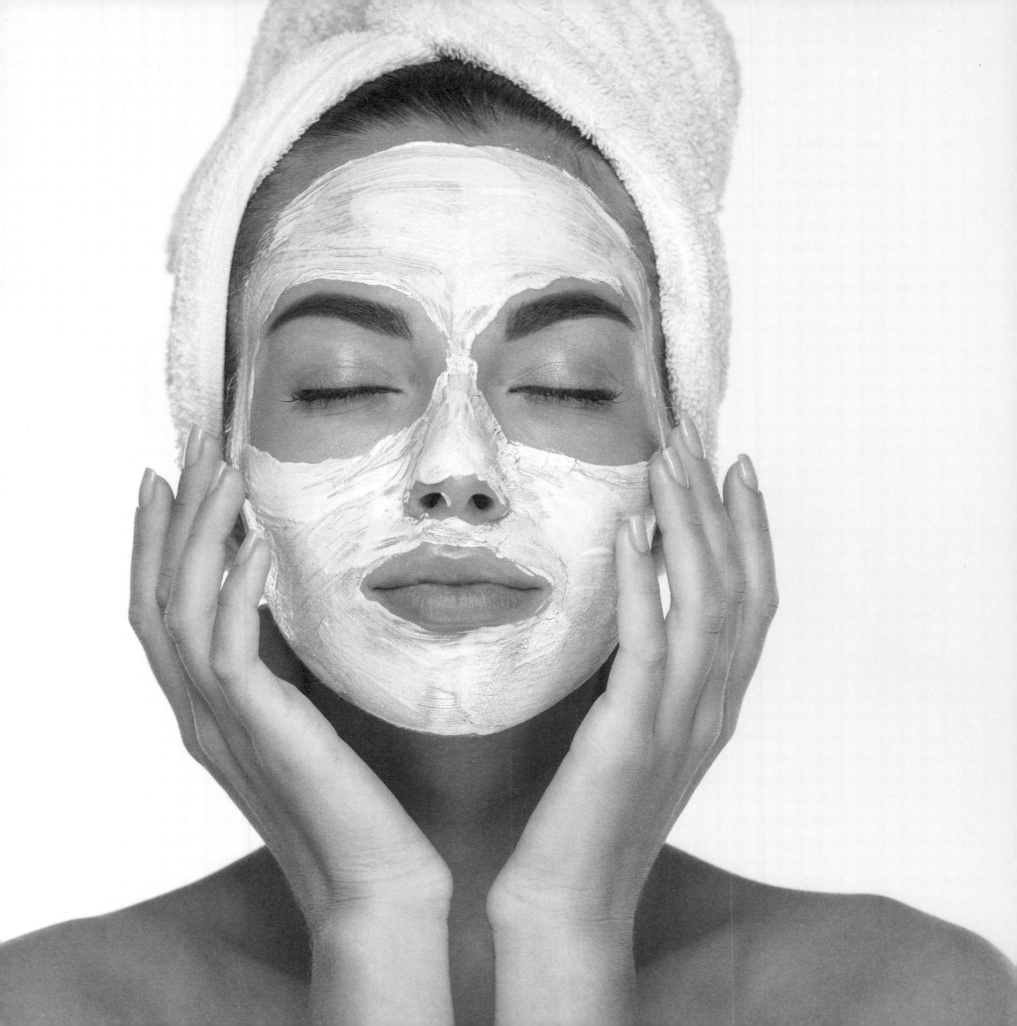

OILY/ACNE PRONE SKIN

Oily skin is characterized by an excess production of oil. The overall pore size is larger and more widespread across the face and has a greater propensity for breakouts. This condition requires more cleansing, exfoliating and treatments. With oily skin, there is a build up of dead skin and oil, creating blockages in the follicle. It seems counterintuitive, but people with oily skin must be careful not to over cleanse and strip the skin. This can lead to irritation and even more oil production, as the skin tries to protect its barrier. While this skin type can be challenging, the silver lining is that those with oily skin tend to show the signs of aging more slowly because the production of oil creates a wonderful layer of protection for the skin.

OILY/ACNE PRONE SKIN CARE ROUTINE

Morning

1. Cleanse with oily- or acne-specific cleanser.
2. Use a toner.
3. Optional: Apply an antioxidant serum, such as vitamin C.
4. Spot treat breakouts, if necessary.
5. Apply oil-free moisturizer.
6. Apply sunscreen (preferably SPF 30, see below).

Note: Look for sunscreens that contain zinc oxide and or titanium dioxide. Try to stay away from chemical sunscreens containing PABA, oxybenzone, octinoxate, homosalate, octisalate, octocrylene and cinnamates, which are ingredients that absorb the sun's UV rays and converts them into heat beneath the skin. This can create irritation and greater inflammation.

Evening

1. Remove all make up and sunscreen.
2. Perform a double cleanse. That means wash and rinse the skin twice.
3. Apply antibacterial toner.
4. Optional (but recommended): Apply a treatment serum, such as Retinol, to promote shedding.
5. Optional: Spot treat breakouts with salicylic acid gel or tea tree oil.
6. Apply oil-free moisturizer.
7. Apply eye cream.

Additionally, try to use a mask twice a week and use ice with inflamed breakouts as necessary. This will help to reduce inflammation.

Note: If you are an athlete and prone to sweat acne, try to cleanse your skin before exercising. If you are outdoors, apply sunscreen thirty minutes prior to your work out and perhaps reapply with a powdered mineral sunscreen as a second layer. If you are exercising inside, try applying a monolaurin gel beforehand and in both cases, double cleanse your skin, as quickly as possible, post workout.

RECOMMENDED INGREDIENTS FOR OILY SKIN

Foam and gel cleansers, anti bacterial toners, masks containing clay, sulfur and anti-inflammatory ingredients. Products containing alpha hydroxy acid (AHA) and beta hydroxy acids (BHA) like salicylic and citric acid can help tremendously.

Diet plays a significant role in skin care so remember to eat a healthy diet and consider an oral supplement containing zinc, vitamins B and vitamin C to help improve skin balance.

COMBINATION SKIN

This skin type requires a little more attention because needs vary. Combination skin can be both oily and normal or oily and dry, simultaneously. The T-Zone area (forehead, nose, chin) usually has a larger follicle size and secretes more oil than other areas of the face. Once again, we are trying to achieve the correct balance of water and oil. Deep pore cleansing is a must and regular exfoliation will help minimize the possibility of a breakout. Water-based products usually work best on this skin type. Follow the routines for oily/acne prone skin but if you feel too dry add a light moisturizer or a ceramide cream. You will have to use your best judgment because your skin condition will vary throughout the month. A licensed esthetician will be very helpful in tailoring a skin care regimen to fit your changing needs.

SENSITIVE SKIN

While sensitive skin is a type, it is also considered a condition. It is usually a result of environmental factors such as pollutants, over exposure to the sun, and stress. The cause can also be one of genetic predisposition. Sensitive skin can be prone to redness and is easily irritated. It is sensitive to heat and sun exposure and can be thin and fragile. Skin sensitivity often increases with age as our production of water and oil diminishes. Be sure you use gentle and calming ingredients at home and in the treatment room. Nourish the skin with humectants and moisturizers and be cognizant of irritants.

SENSITIVE SKIN ROUTINE

Morning

1. Rinse with warm water.
2. Use a gentle toner.
3. Optional: Apply an antioxidant serum, my favorite is a vitamin C serum, with or without vitamin E.
4. Apply moisturizer.
5. Apply eye cream.
6. Apply sunscreen (broad spectrum UVA/UVB with at least SPF 30).

Note: As with sensitive skin, look for sunscreens that contain zinc oxide and or titanium dioxide. Try to stay away from chemical sunscreens containing PABA, oxybenzone, octinoxate, homosalate, octisalate, octocrylene and cinnamates, which are ingredients that absorb the sun's UV rays and convert them into heat beneath the skin. This can create irritation and greater inflammation.

Evening

1. Remove make-up and sunscreen (try a miceller water or oil cleansers).
2. Double cleanse with a gentle cream cleanser.
3. Use a gentle toner.
4. Optional: Apply nutrient-rich serum to help repair barrier.
5. Apply hydrating moisturizer.
6. Apply eye cream.

The goal with sensitive and sensitized skin is to calm and cool. Ingredients to keep in mind are aloe vera, allantoin, azulene, chamomile and licorice. Be mindful of irritants such as fragrances, color agents, essential oils and preservatives.

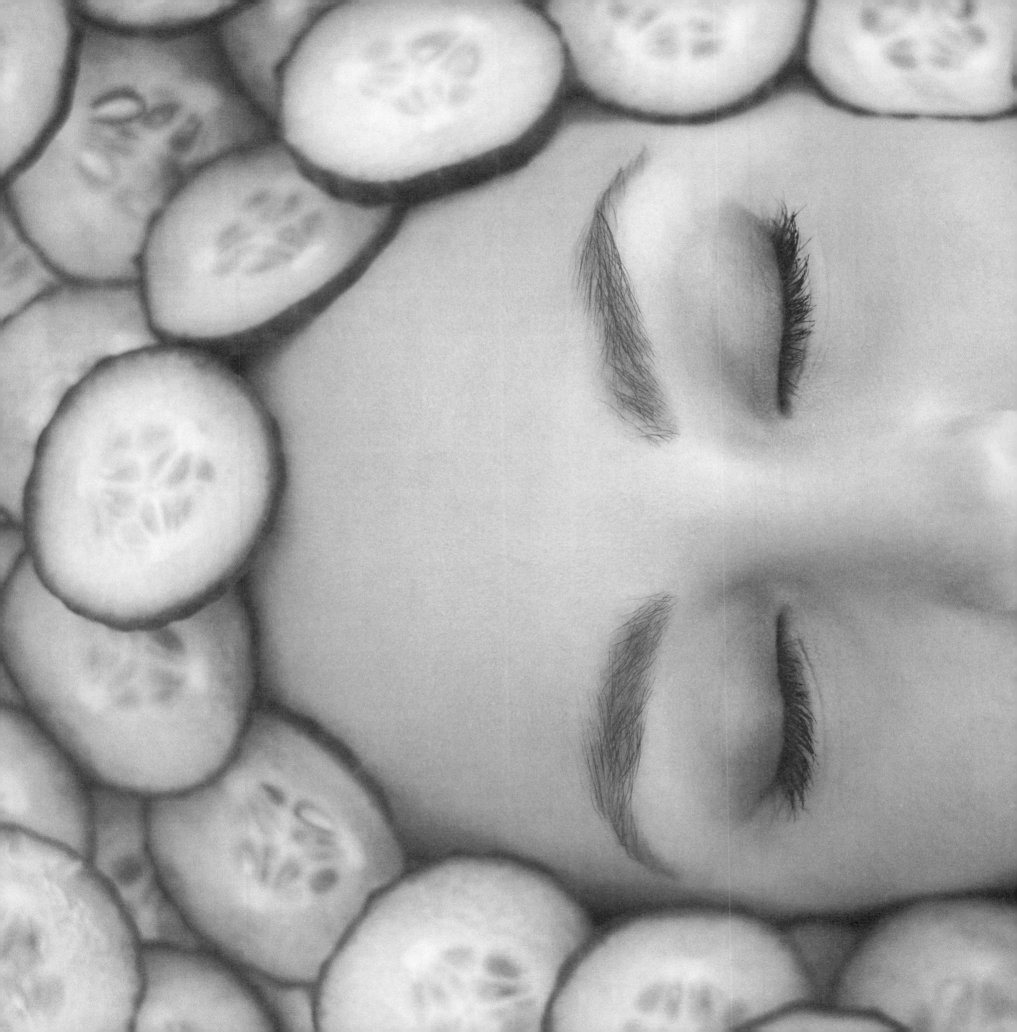

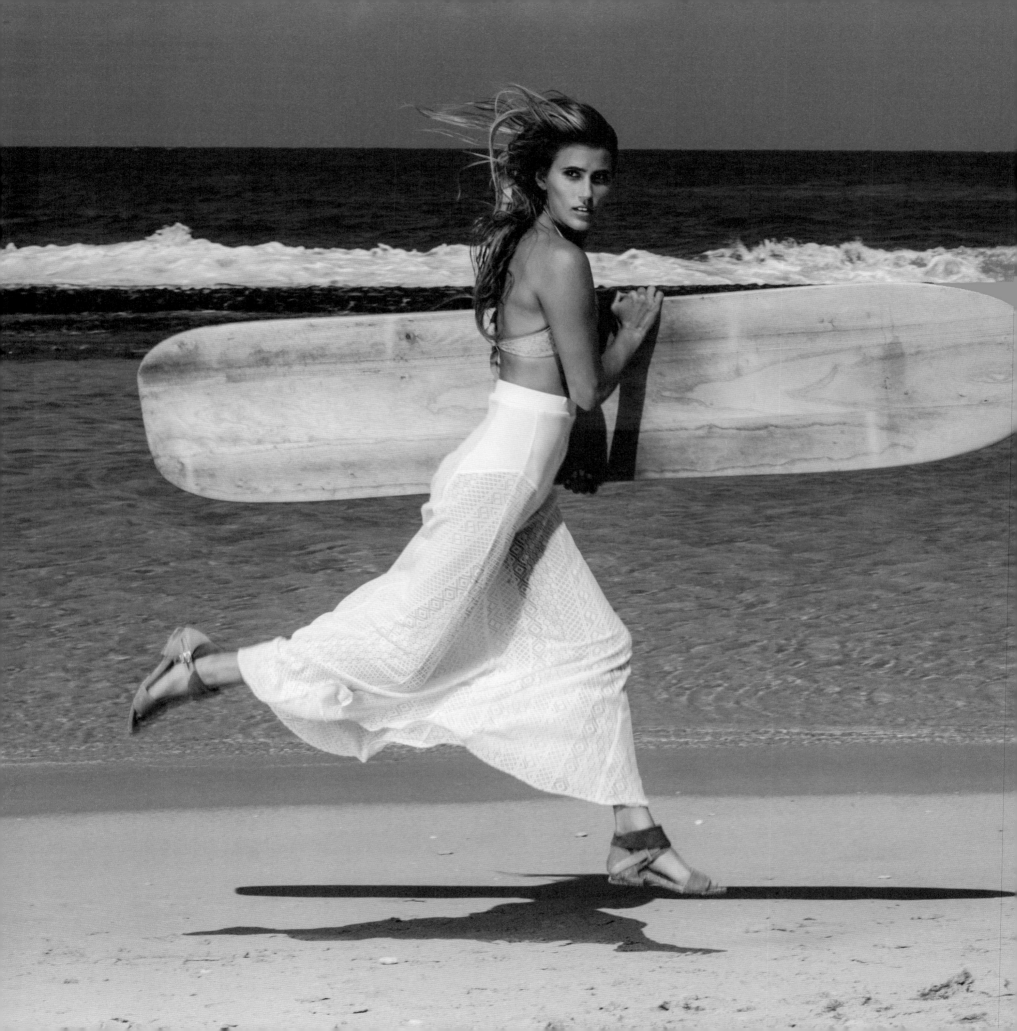

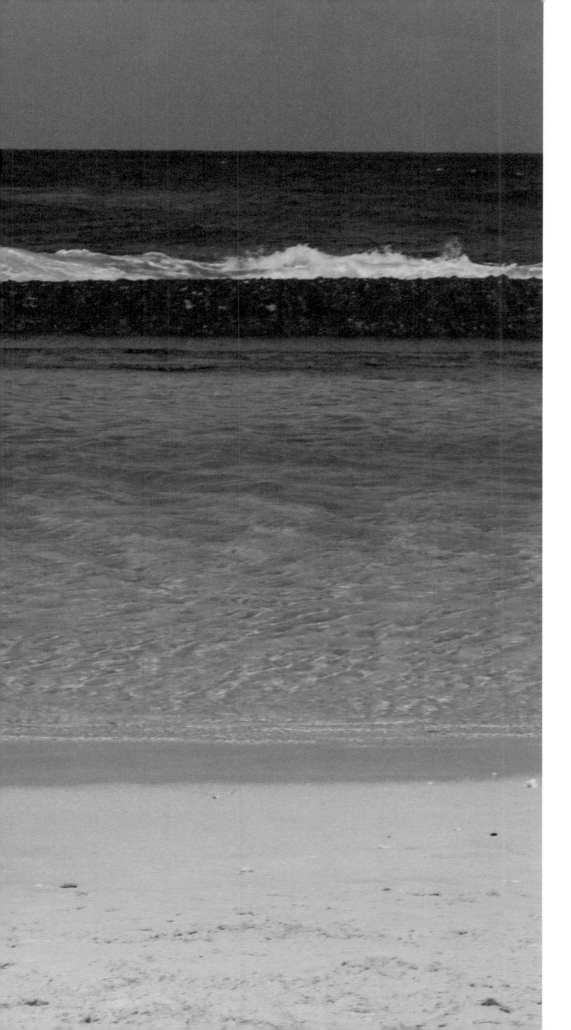

Part 4

EXERCISE & SLEEP

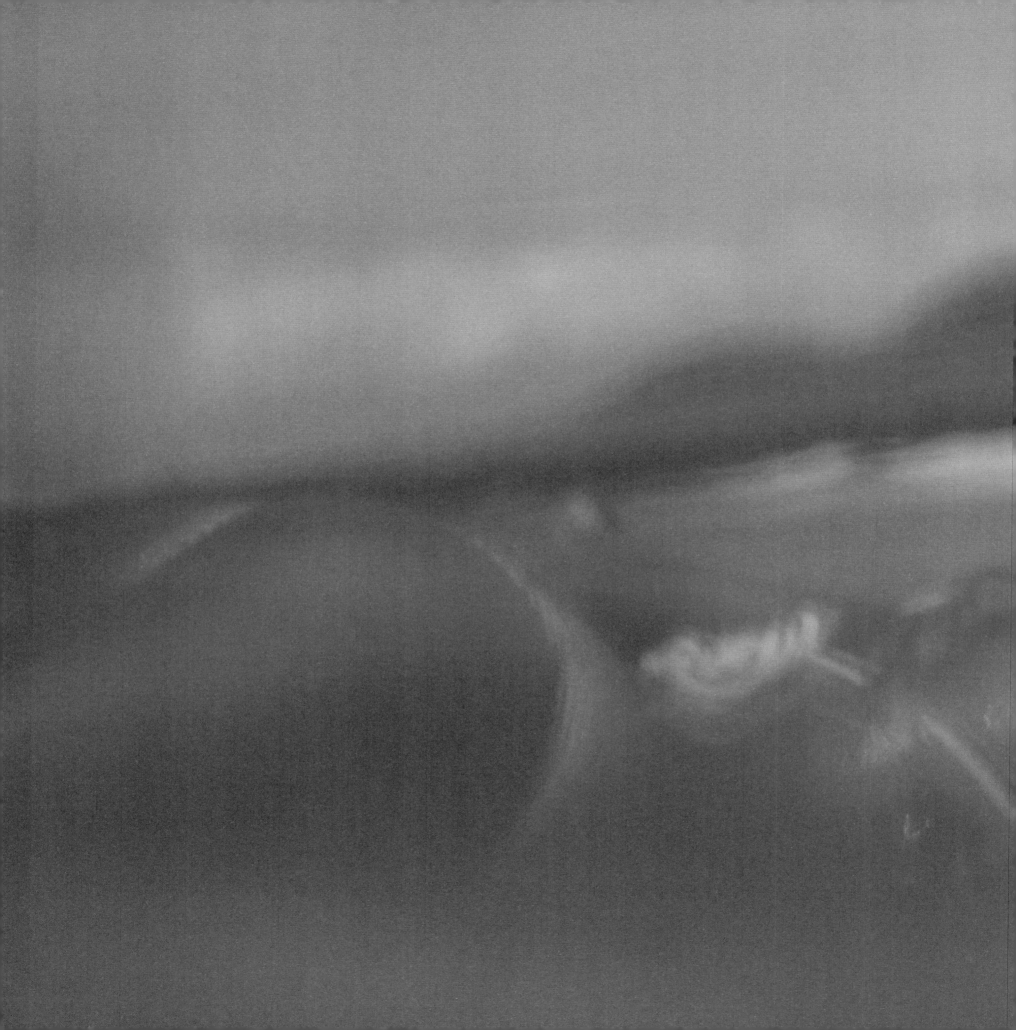

AMAZING ATHLETES

Photographic Collection

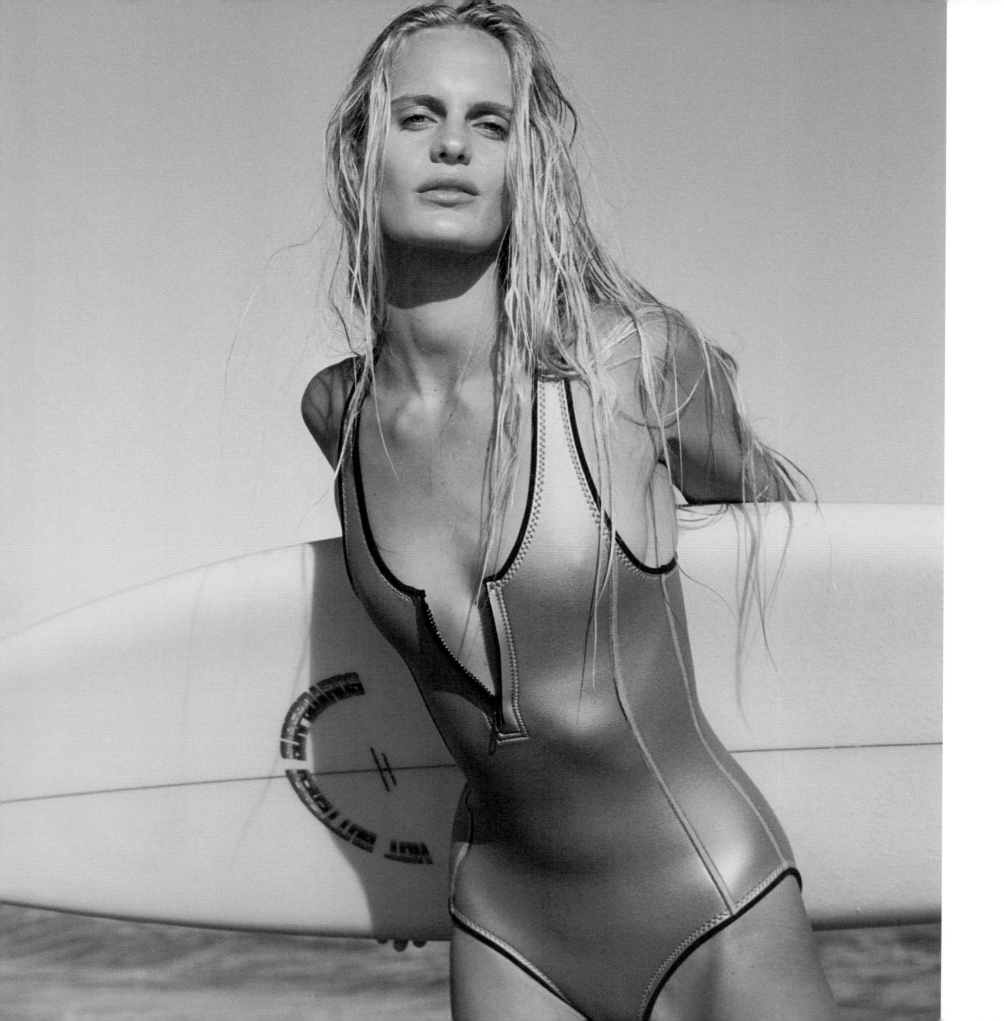

"Yes Hanalei, like the bay. It means moon crescent. It is a special name, that I am very grateful to have. I am from Tahiti, where dreams become reality."

"Surfing came as a natural thing in my life, like a blessing from the Gods. I remember my brother and I standing up on my dad's boards, spending hours in the water, like dolphins in their element. Now it is my life, because everything revolves around waves, swells, new spots, fins, boards, leashes and wax. It's a passion, a passion that I share with mother nature."

Hanalei Reponty
Mermaid, model, surfer and
founder of Abysse Swimwear

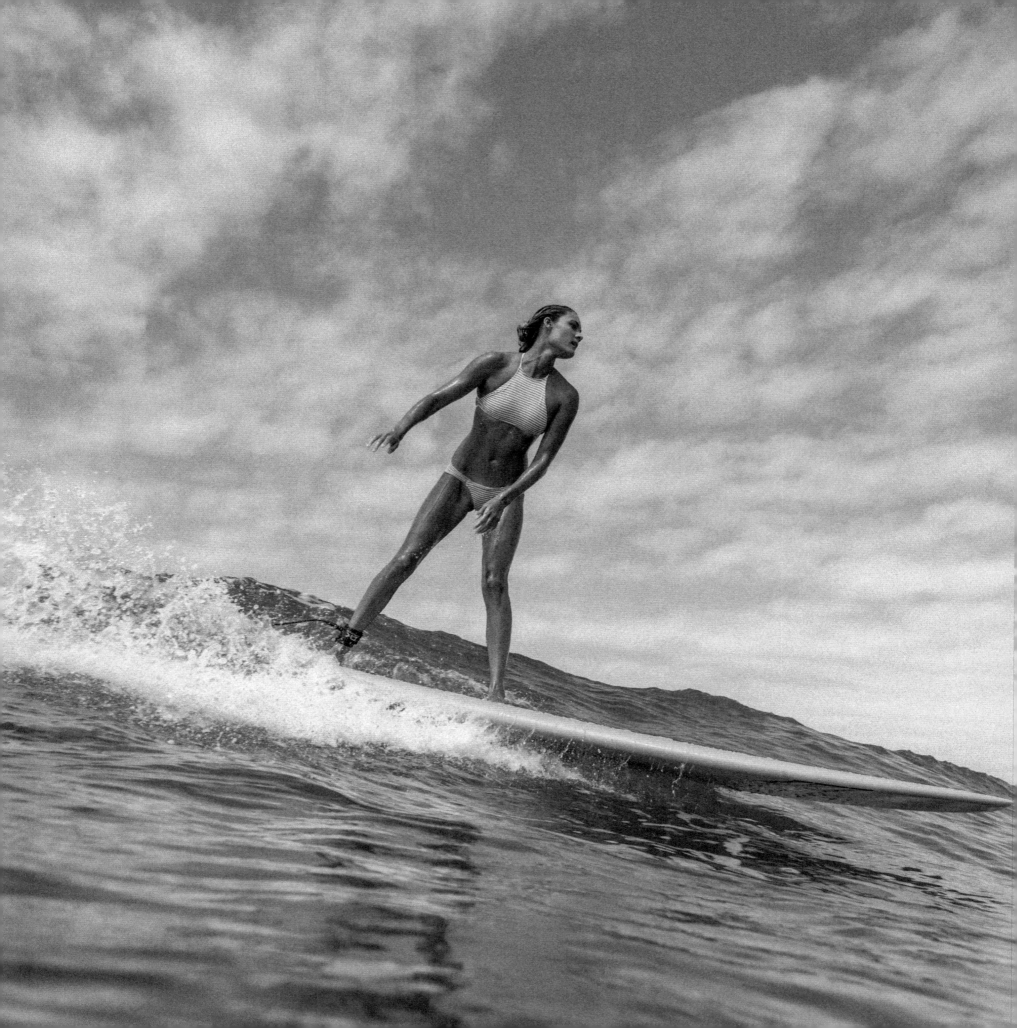

"To have good health of the mind, body and soul is a privilege to be preserved by cultivating a healthy lifestyle within ourselves and with others."

Kelly Gallaher
Surfer and student

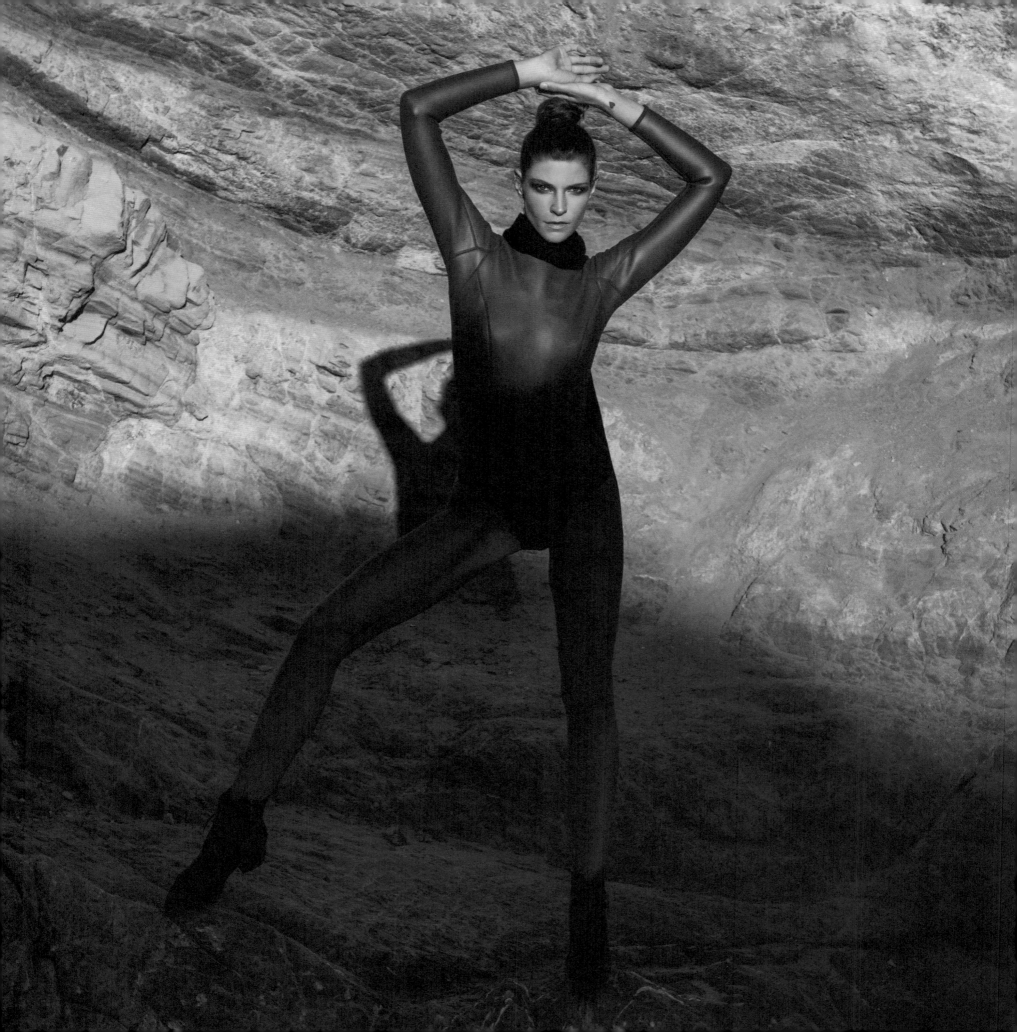

"**Wellness** is a mindset. If you have a positive one you will find happiness most anywhere. There are infinite ways to get into a positive outlook. Laugh, play, meditate, do what you love. Find your thing and don't let anyone or anything stop you, but know the foundation will always be fragile without real, unprocessed foods and intense exercise at whatever level you are. Even if you're a couch potato playing video games, just jump up and down on that sofa until you pass out like a **rock star.**"

Aleksandra Rastovic
Producer, director, ocean activist and mermaid

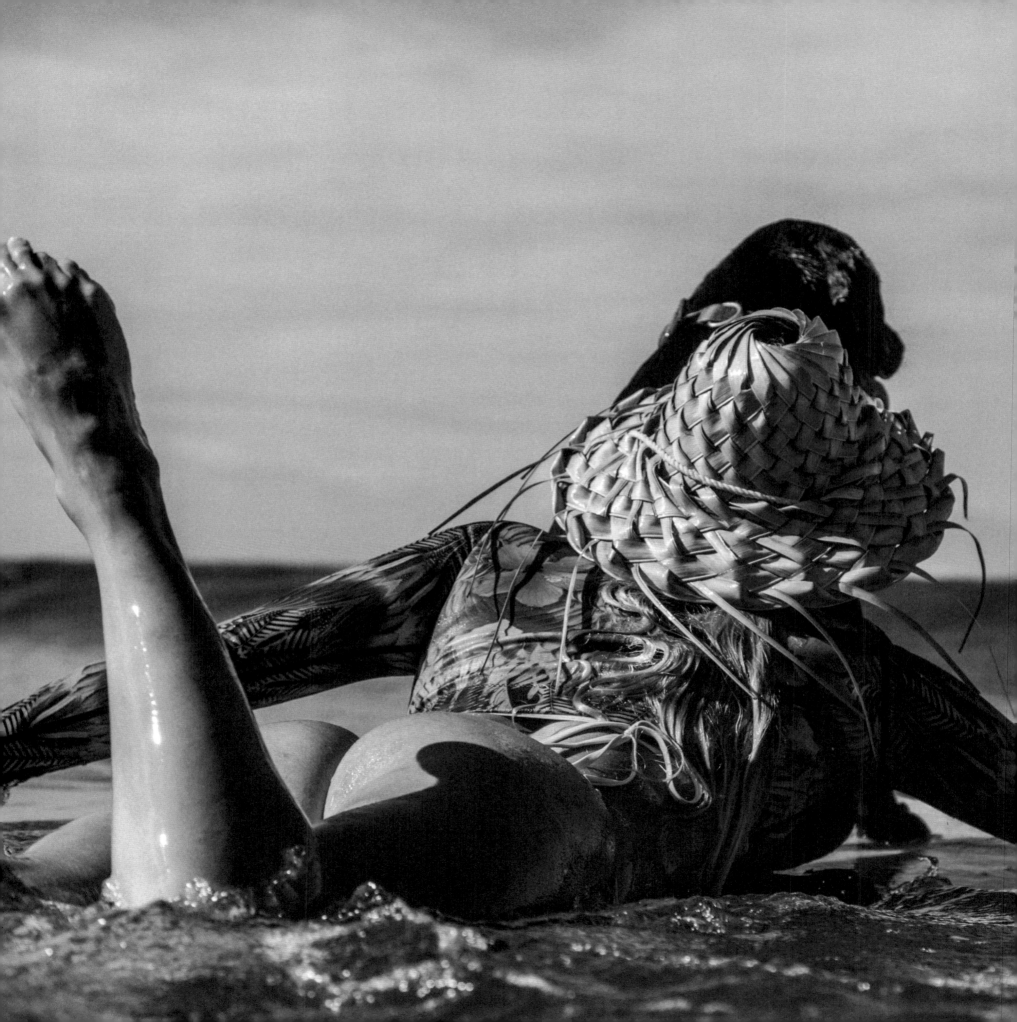

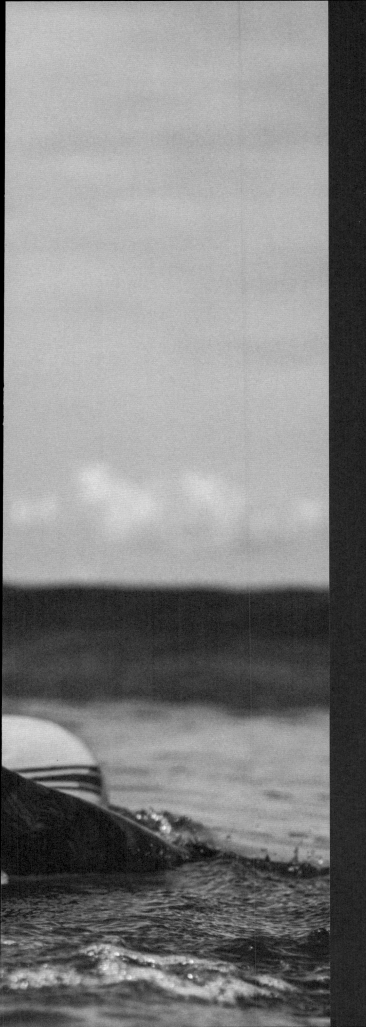

"No matter what's going on in my life; emotionally and physically, the one thing I can always count on to spark the flame in me, is jumping into the ocean. It's cleansing, making it apparent to me that the only thing that really matters is being in the present moment, and receiving it for exactly what it is, a present. To me that's the ultimate wellness."

Ashley Baxter
Model, pro water athlete

"The best way to live a healthy life is to feed your body healthy food, feed your mind positive thoughts and get moving as much as possible."

April Mancuso Reynolds
Mama, wife, doctor, wellness entrepreneur, skier and water girl

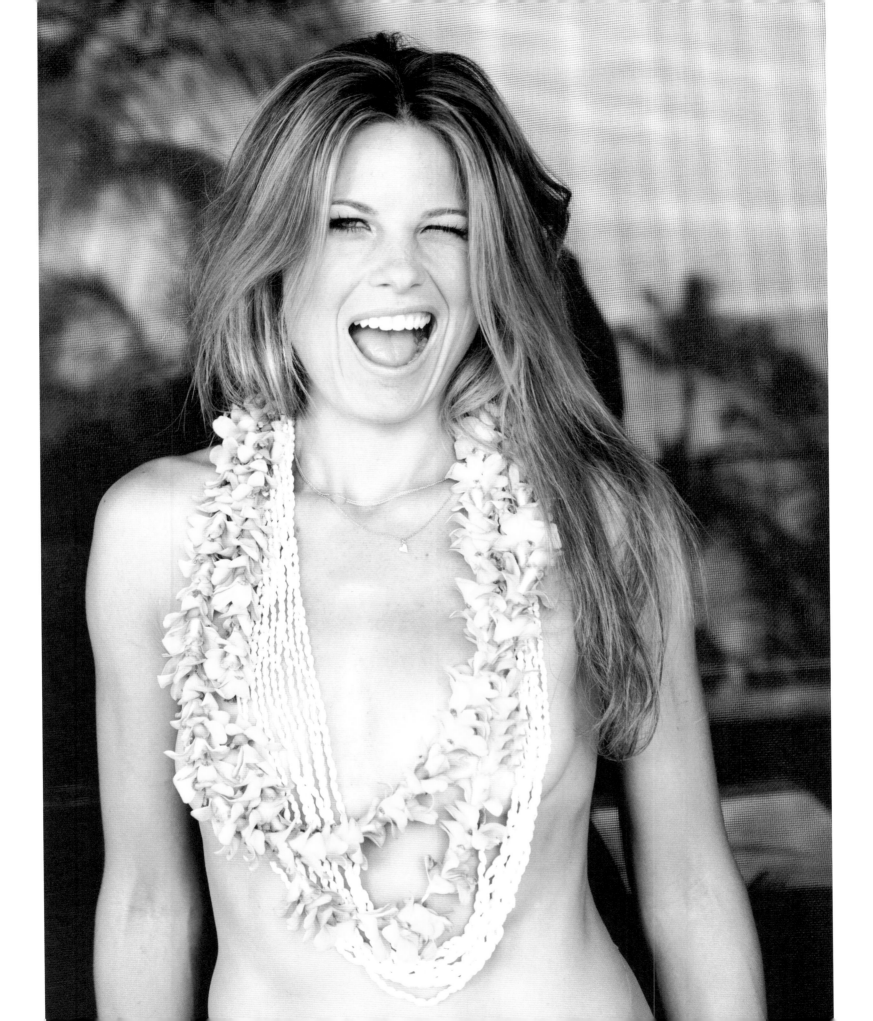

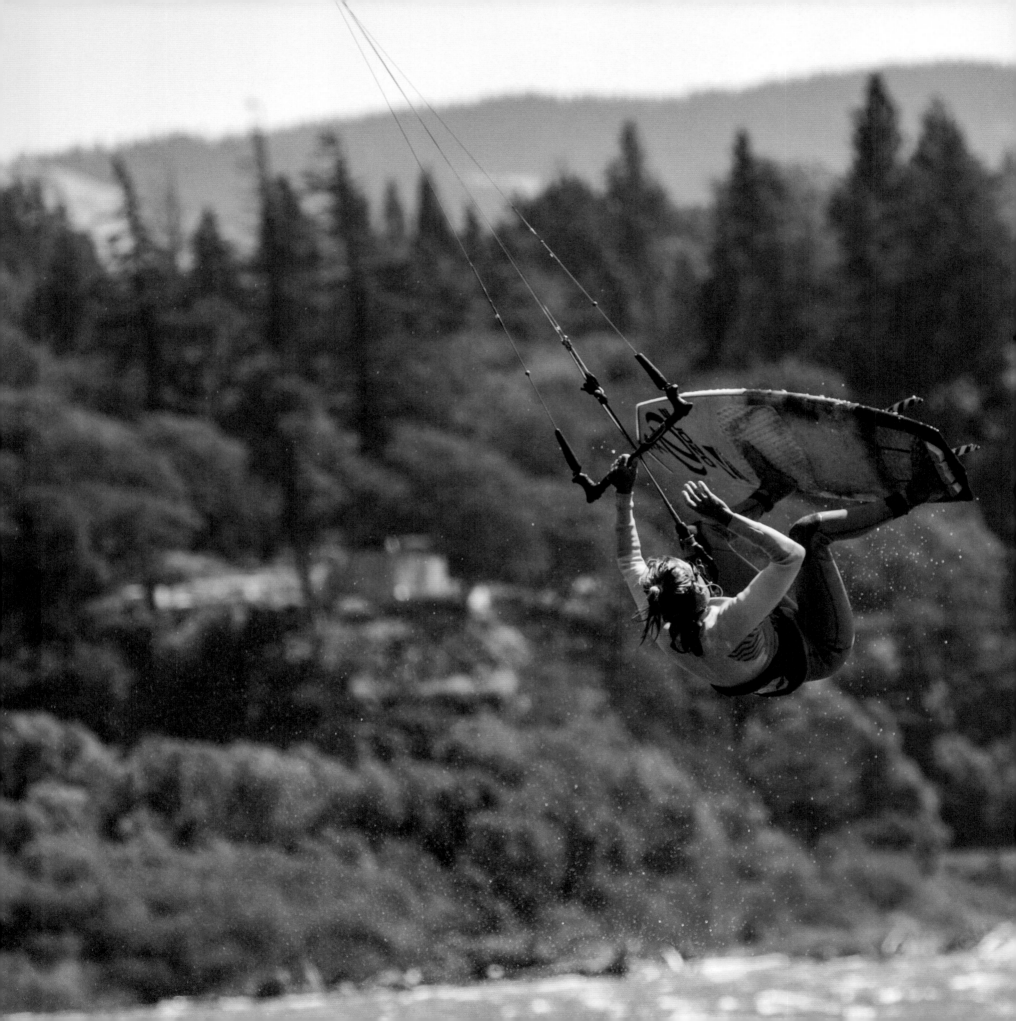

"To be honest, I spend almost as much time in the air as I do in or on the water, yet it's the water that gives me the power to fly. When I am kitesurfing I feel as if I am a child, dancing, splashing and giggling. Supreme athleticism is effort-less. It is only when I touch back on land that I feel gravity and the weight of my years."

Cynthia 'Cynbad' Brown
Pro kitesurfer

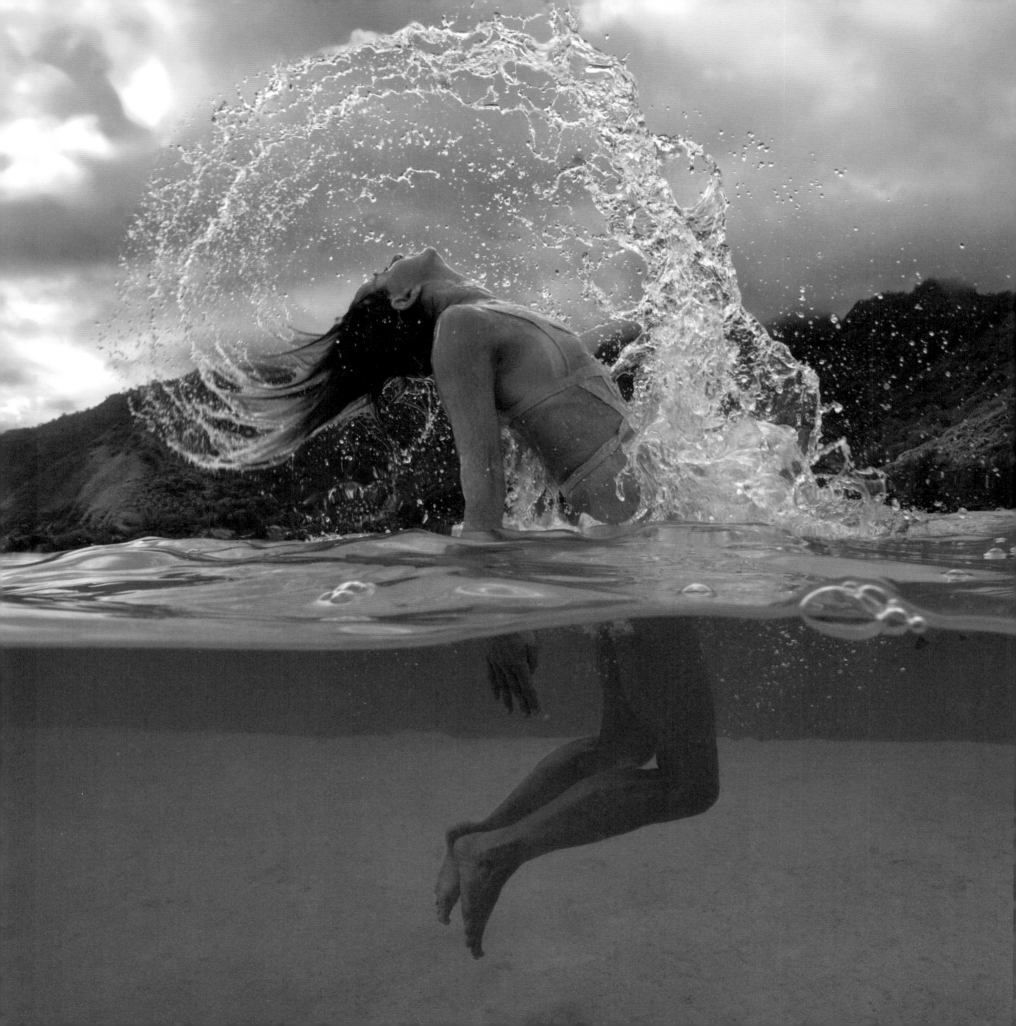

"It's almost like I have two lives. Half of me is a mermaid (I am a Pisces) and the other half of me, I think belongs on land. I am at my best when I come out of the water wearing a huge smile and the rest of the day is but a dream for me. This is truly my path to wellness. What is yours?"

Neely Mack
Mermaid, mama, co-founder of Junbesi Group, fashion designer, creator of Project You, skier, surfer, runner and tennis player

"After years of high-school, college and professional running - the goal was always to win. As a mother of four, I come in fifth now, not first anymore. Fifth place never felt so good."

Clara Horowitz Peterson
Five-time NEAA all-American, 2.35 marathoner and mother of four

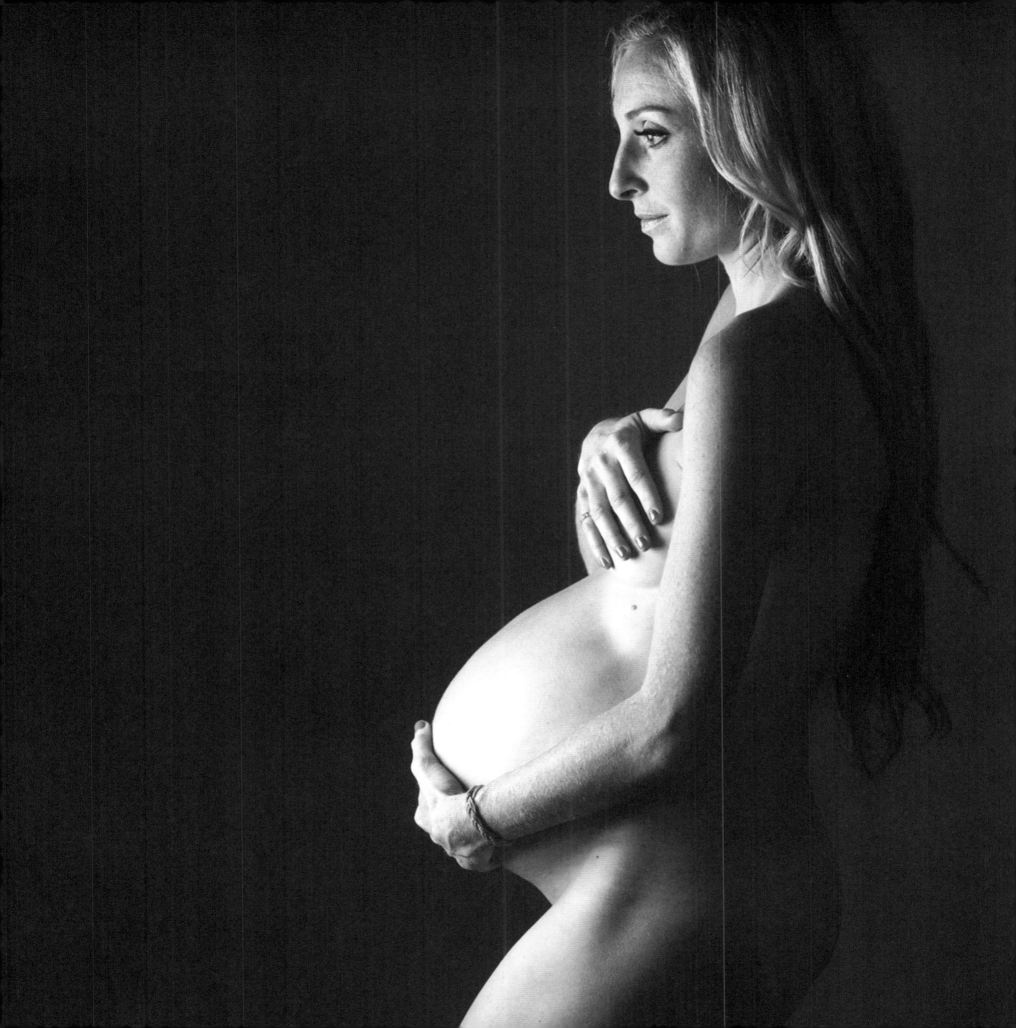

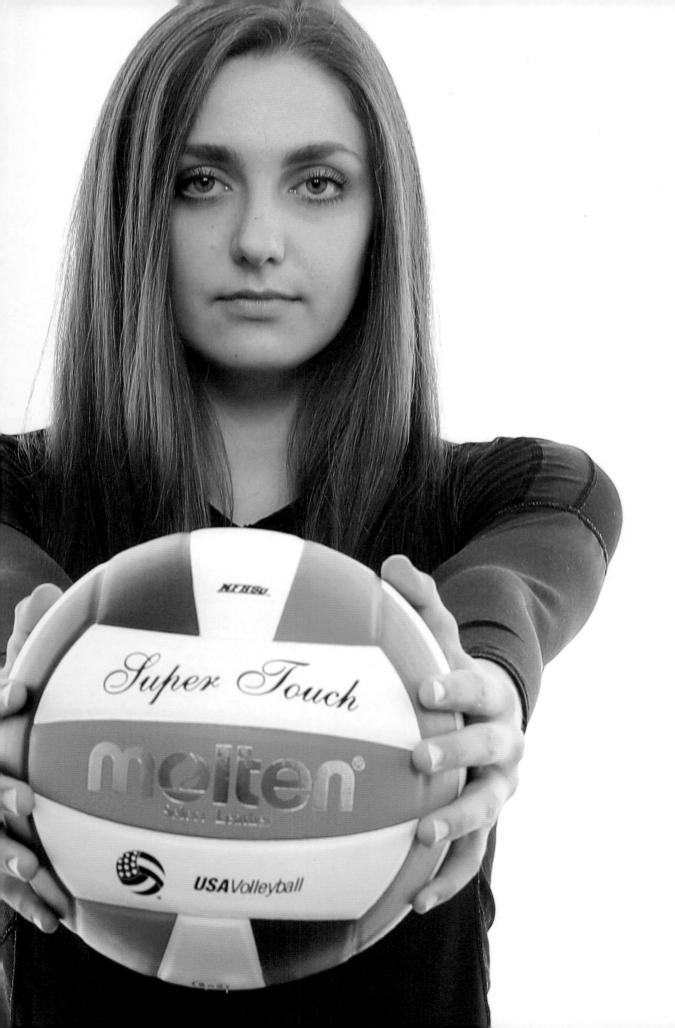

"Wellness is consciously maintaining a healthy body and mind while actively attempting to make positive impact on our environment and the people in it."

McKenzie Cooke
Student and Yale volleyball player

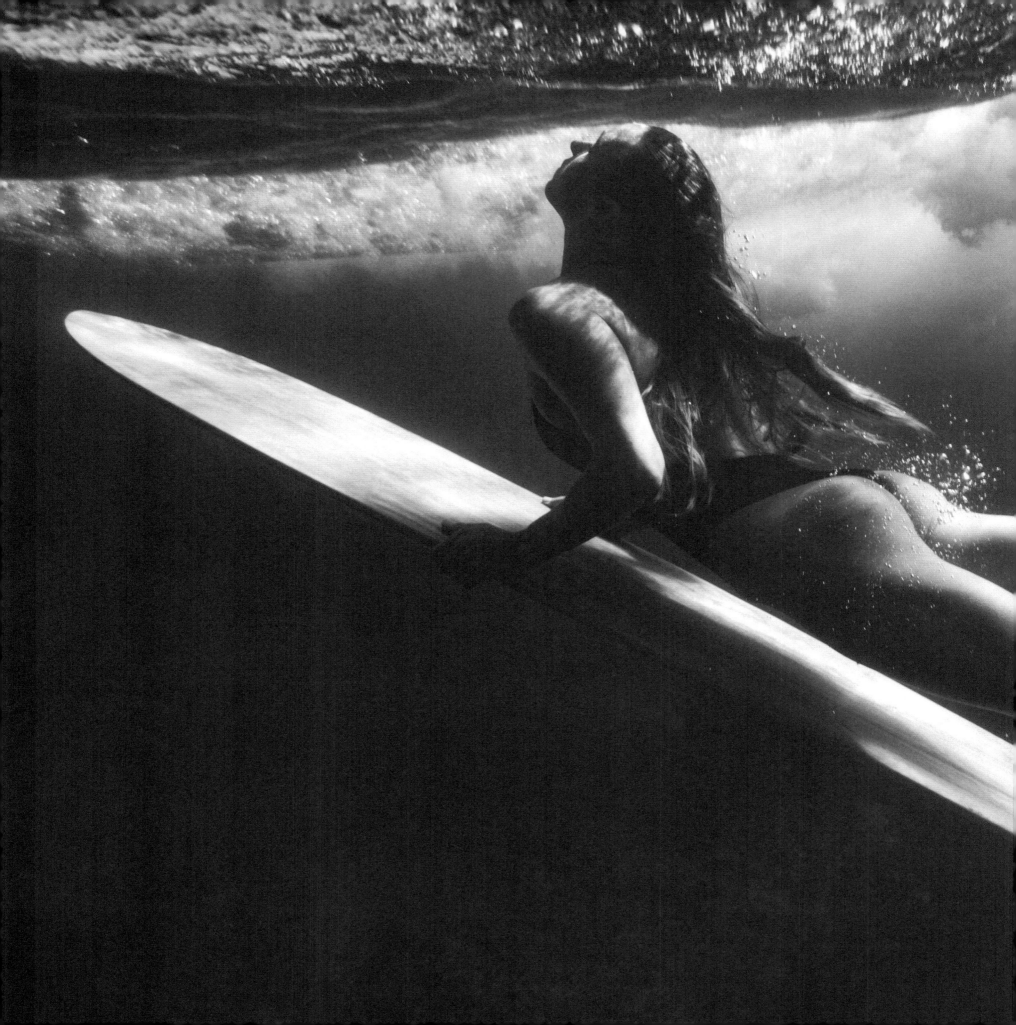

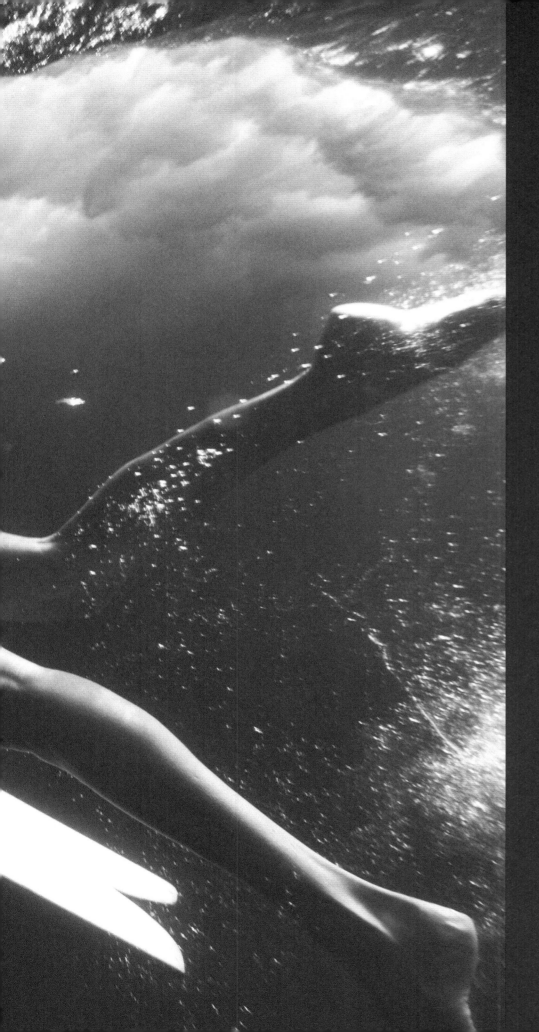

"I try to eat a rainbow a day, for my health is my greatest wealth. I put myself in nature every day, I feel the earth beneath my bare feet and take a deep breath. I let the salt kiss my lips and the sun warm my soul. I remind myself to be grateful and to be by myself."

Sarah Stein
Surfer

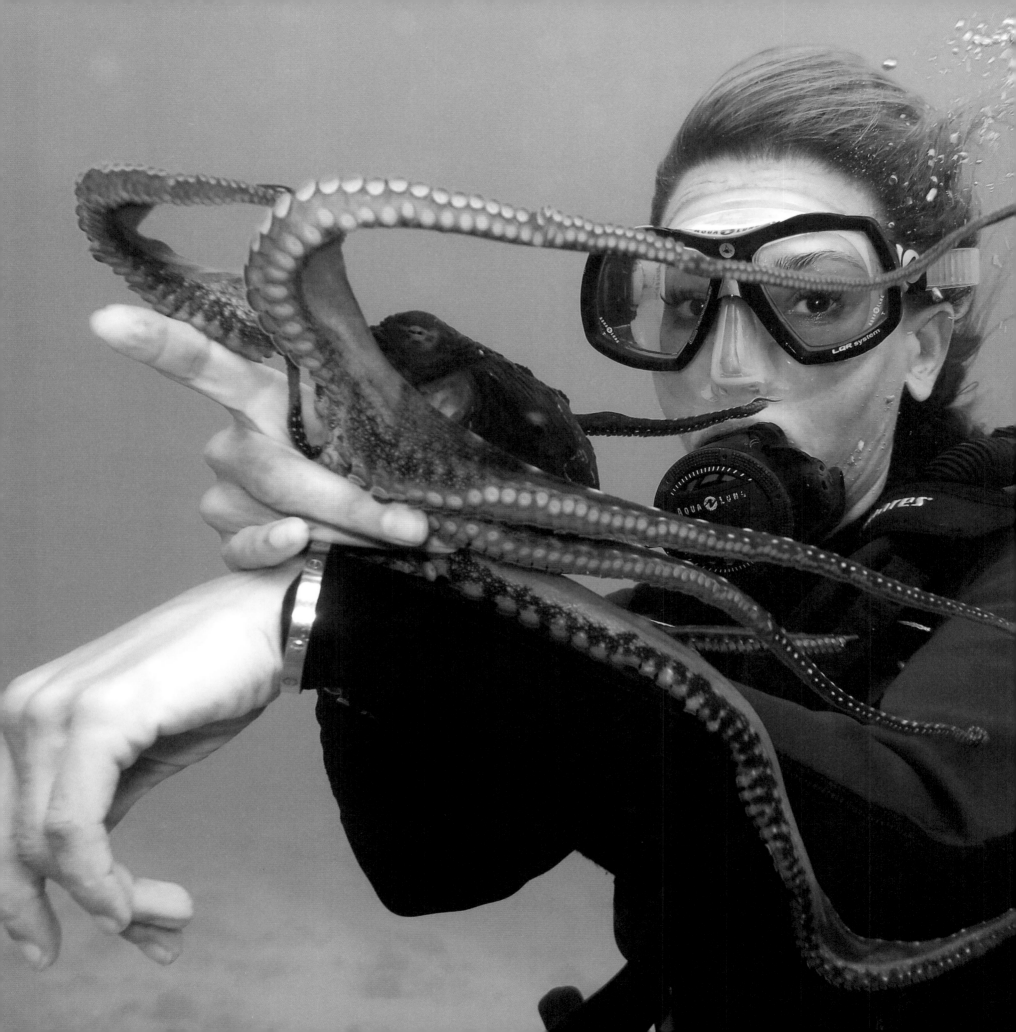

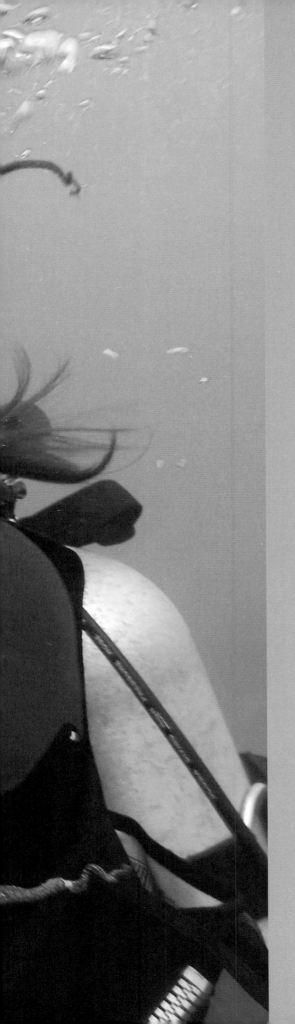

"**Wellness is the constant evolution of one's body, mind and soul toward optimal health.**"

Ginger Robin
Mom and scuba diver

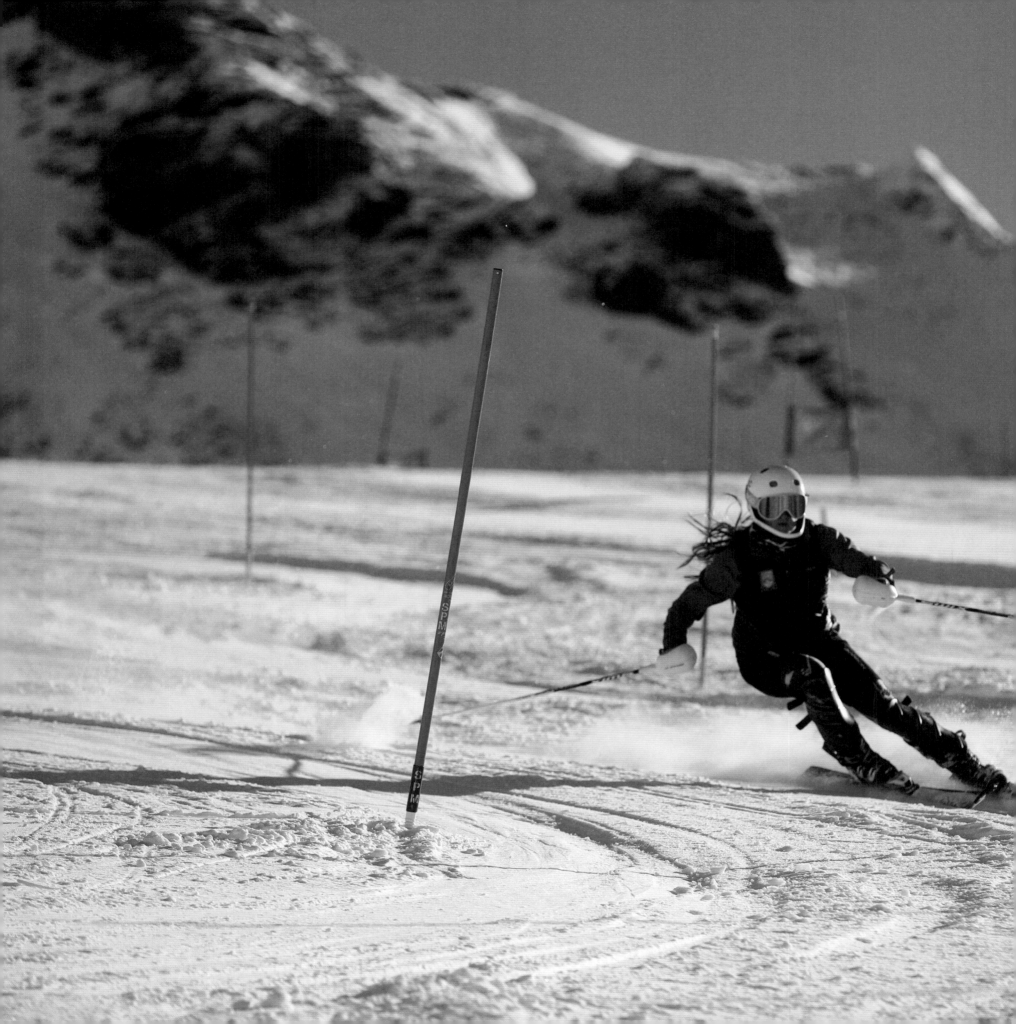

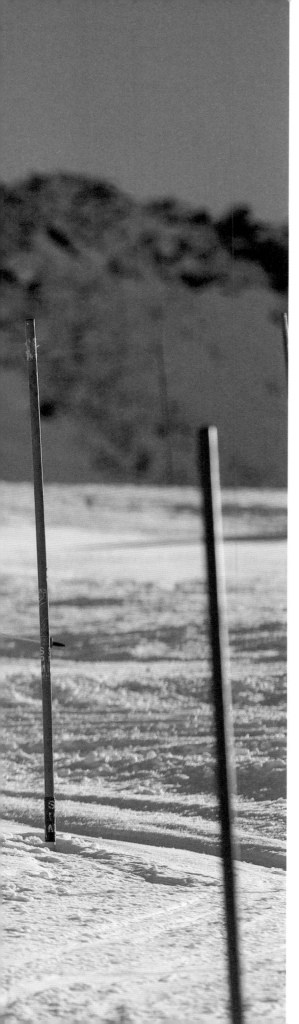

"Skiing is the perfect balance between passion, adversity and gratification. There is no better feeling than free skiing on a powder day or carving a GS turn. Skiing at high speeds is a unique intangible experience but I also love the challenge of working to be cleaner and faster!"

Daphne James
Student and alpine ski racer

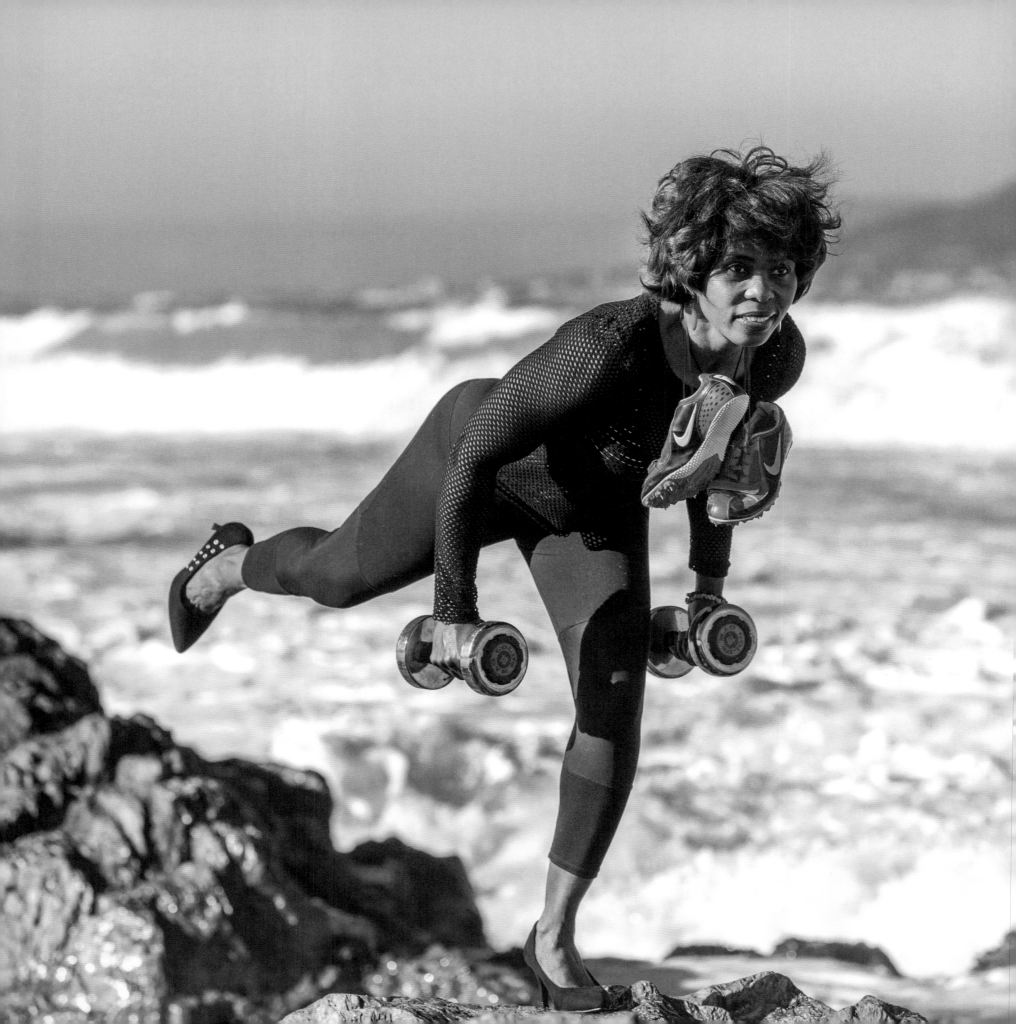

"From earning a living racing the clock to the lowest possible time I could sprinting from point A to B, which I could only achieve through being strong, fit and well balanced mentally, emotionally, spiritually and physically. I now know that every breath I take must be sustained through certain traits and behavior and some level of effort to maintain and prolong my existence. This evoked my intellectual depth about how the human body functions. I have a deeper sense of purpose, need and desire to have great energy, happiness, clarity, positive perspective, hope and strength for me and those around me.

Health and Wellness is the pillar of human existence, which all humanity should consciously strive for and be inspired to pursue for a greater sense of purpose and life fulfillment."

Winneth Dube

2002 Commonwealth Games semi-finalist, World Champion quarter-finalist, Olympian, Zimbabwe National Record Holder (in 60m, 200m indoor and 100m, 200m outdoor), 10 years military service (AFZ), computer programmer, wellness and fitness coach and motivational speaker

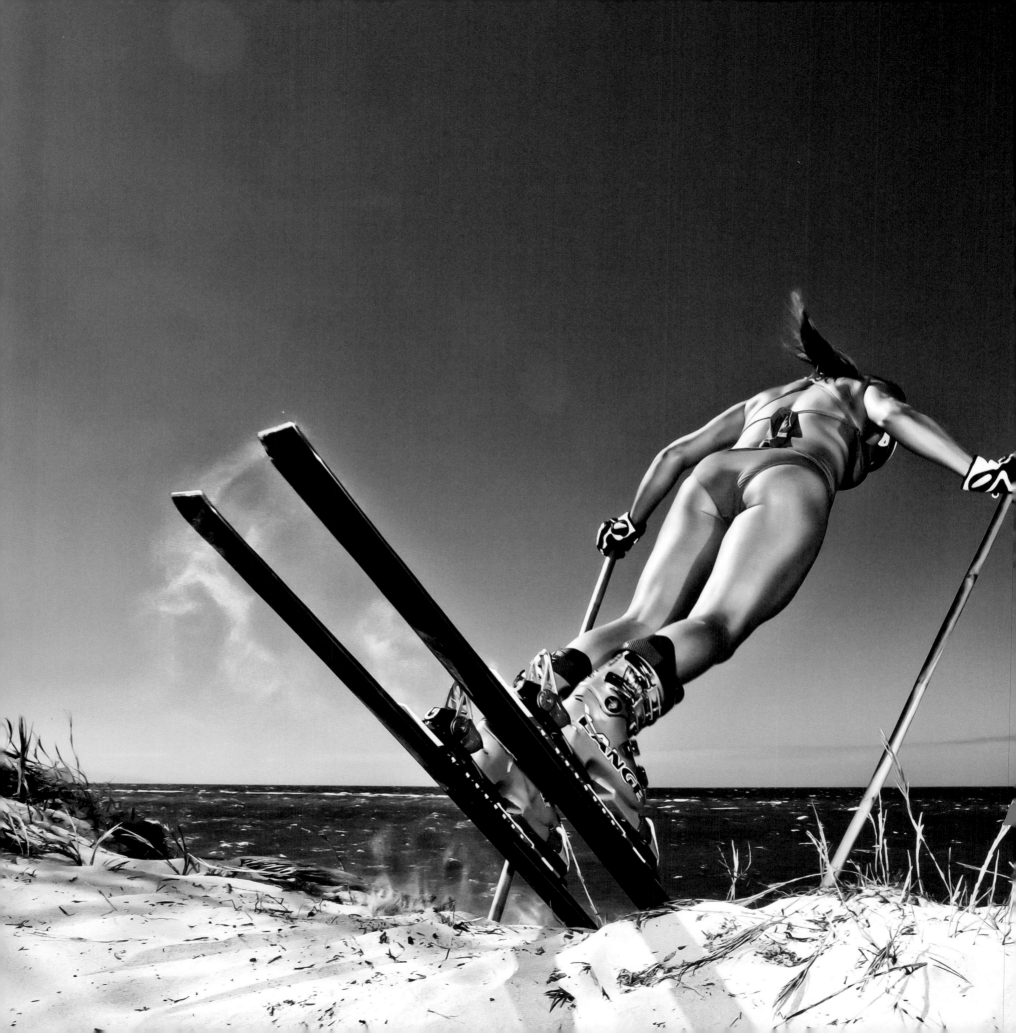

"**Health is freedom to enjoy every moment of life with 100 percent of your energy.**"

Julia Mancuso
*American World Cup alpine ski racer,
Olympic gold medalist, two-time Olympic
silver medalist and bronze medalist*

"Being in tune with my feelings and enjoying the smallest moments in life."

Olivia Cooke
Student and competitive swimmer

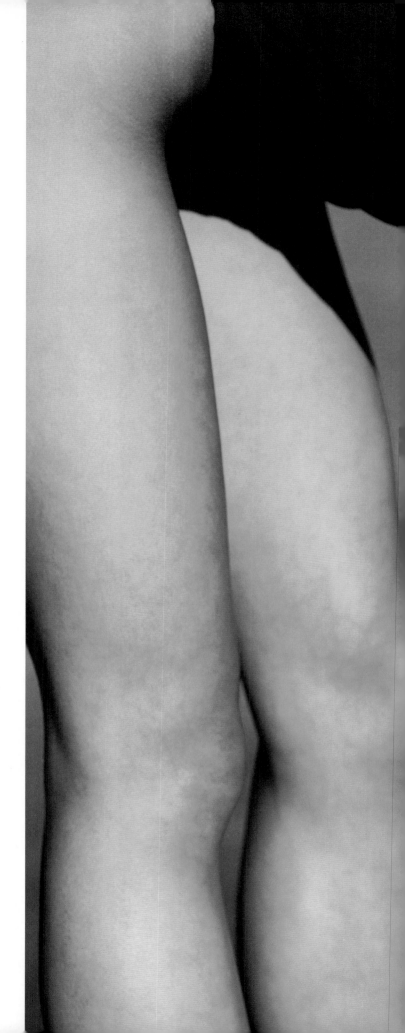

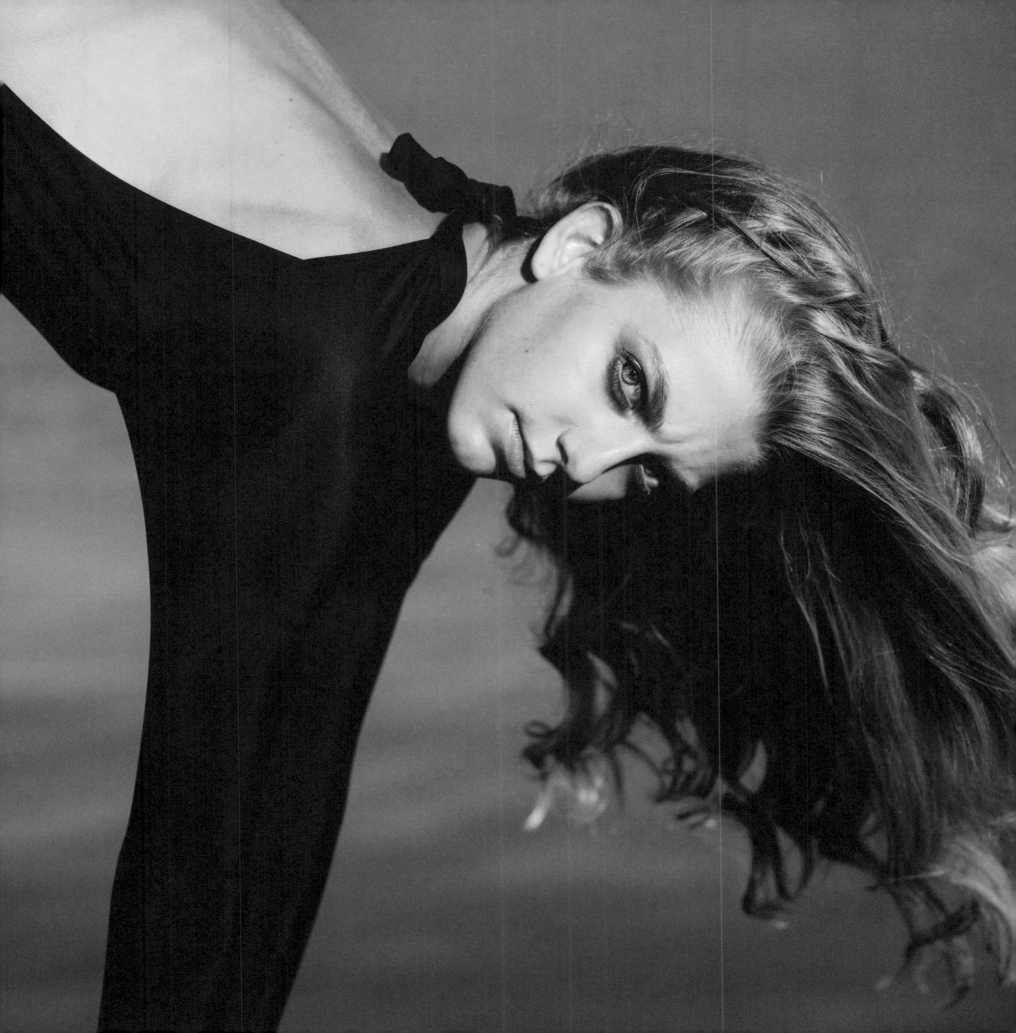

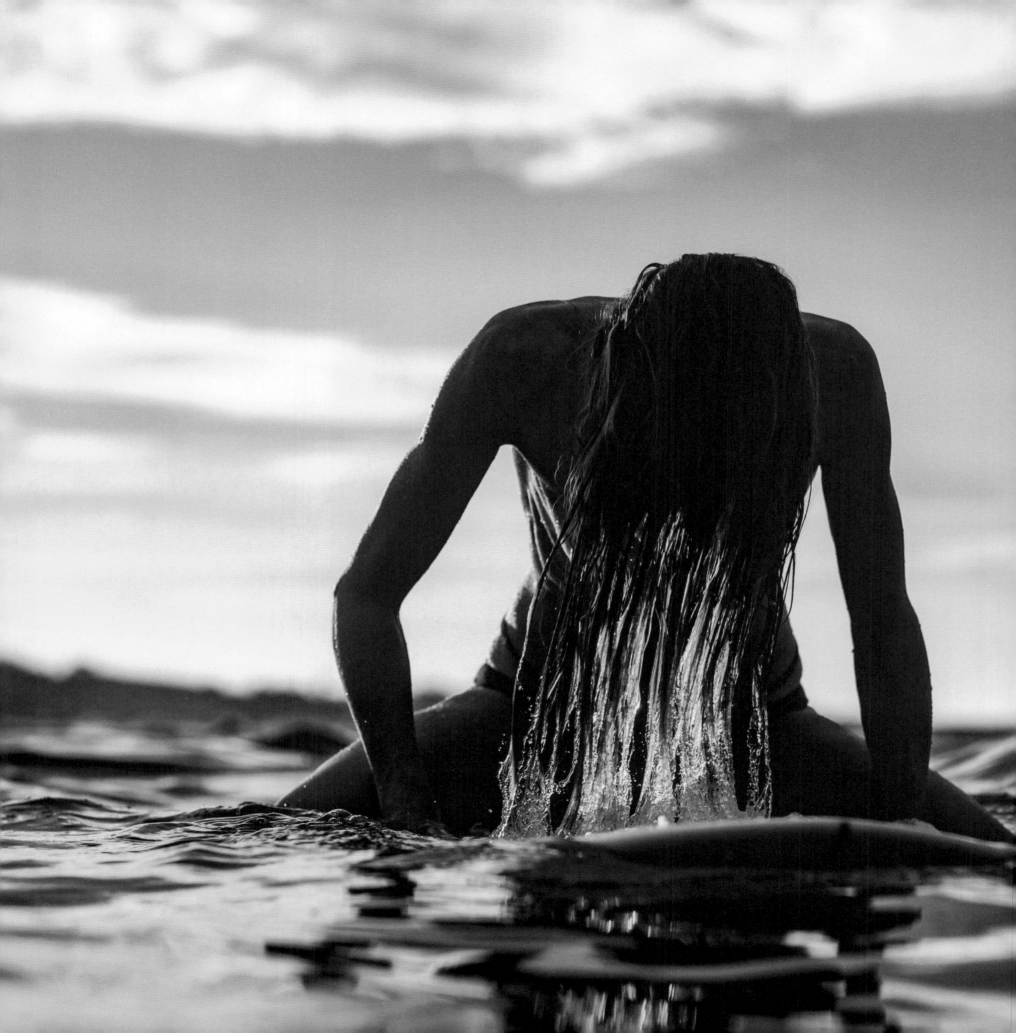

"Embracing Mother Nature in all her elements through skiing, swimming, biking, running, surfing…is a feeling of independence and freedom. Doing anything outdoors makes me feel free, whole and complete with nature."

Sandy Holbrook James
Mermaid, mama, health coach,
triathlete and skier

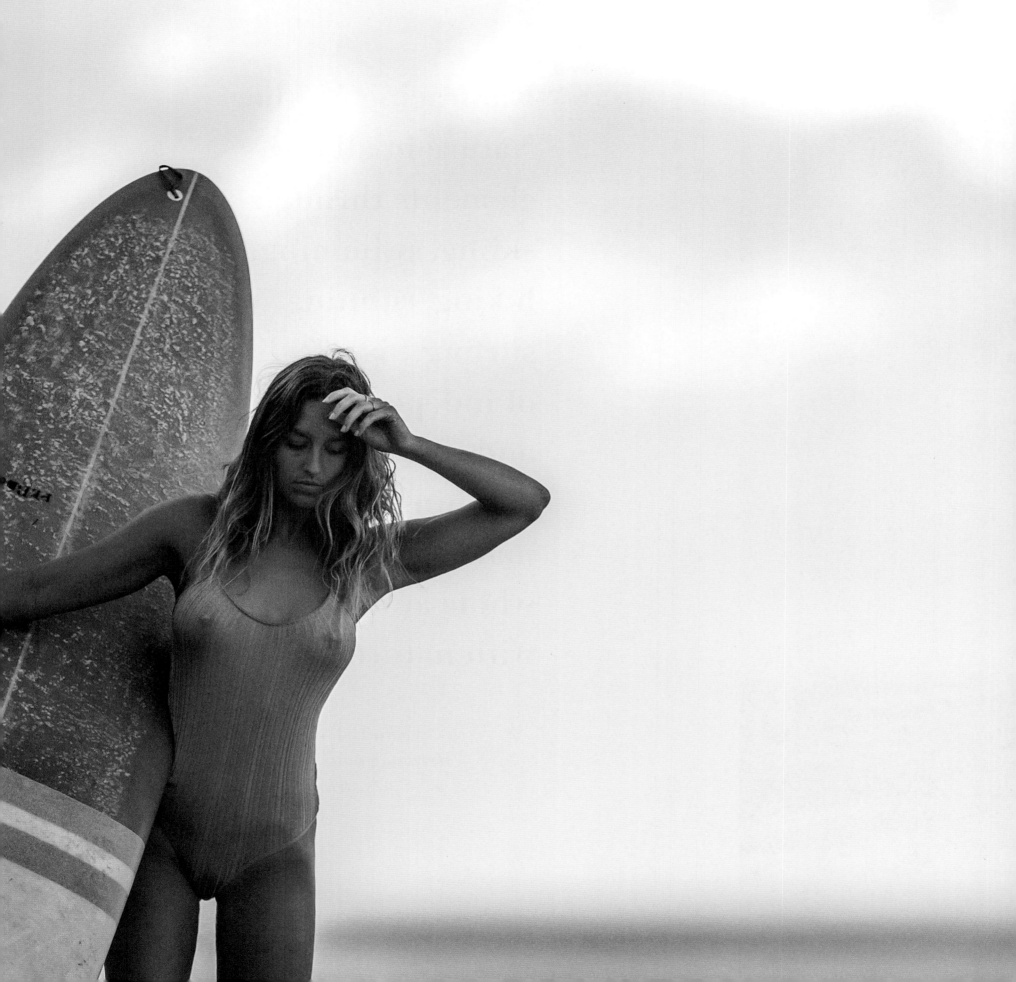

"A healthy spirit in a healthy body – this is the key to happiness and wellbeing."

Alice Arutkin
Pro windsurfer

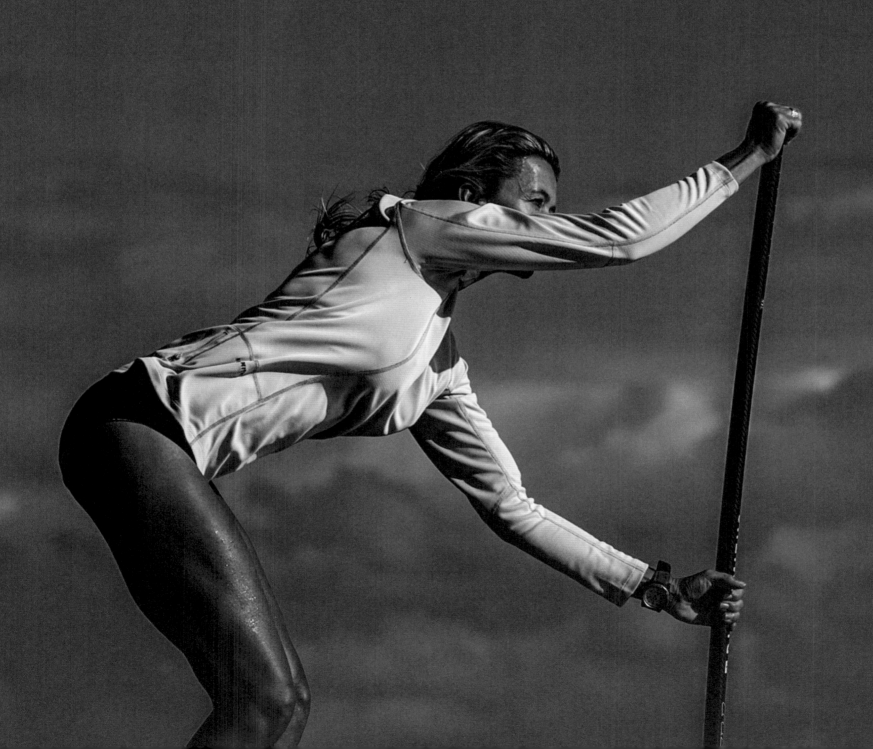

"Every ocean adventure is the way I feed my soul. I respect and accept the challenges that rise in the waves as the wind carries me swiftly."

Suzie Cooney
Mermaid, pro stand-up paddler trainer and owner of Suzie Trains Maui

"Running makes me feel free."

Lucie James
Student, competitive runner

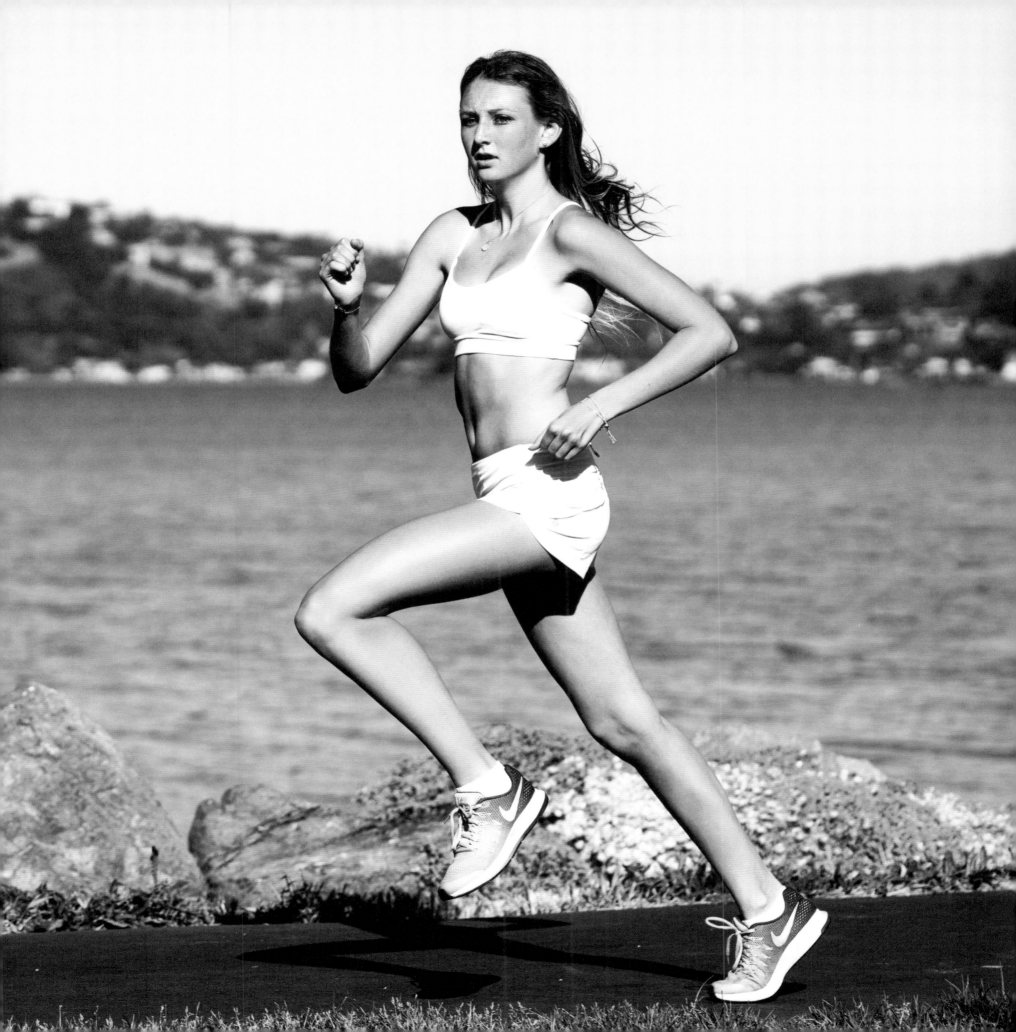

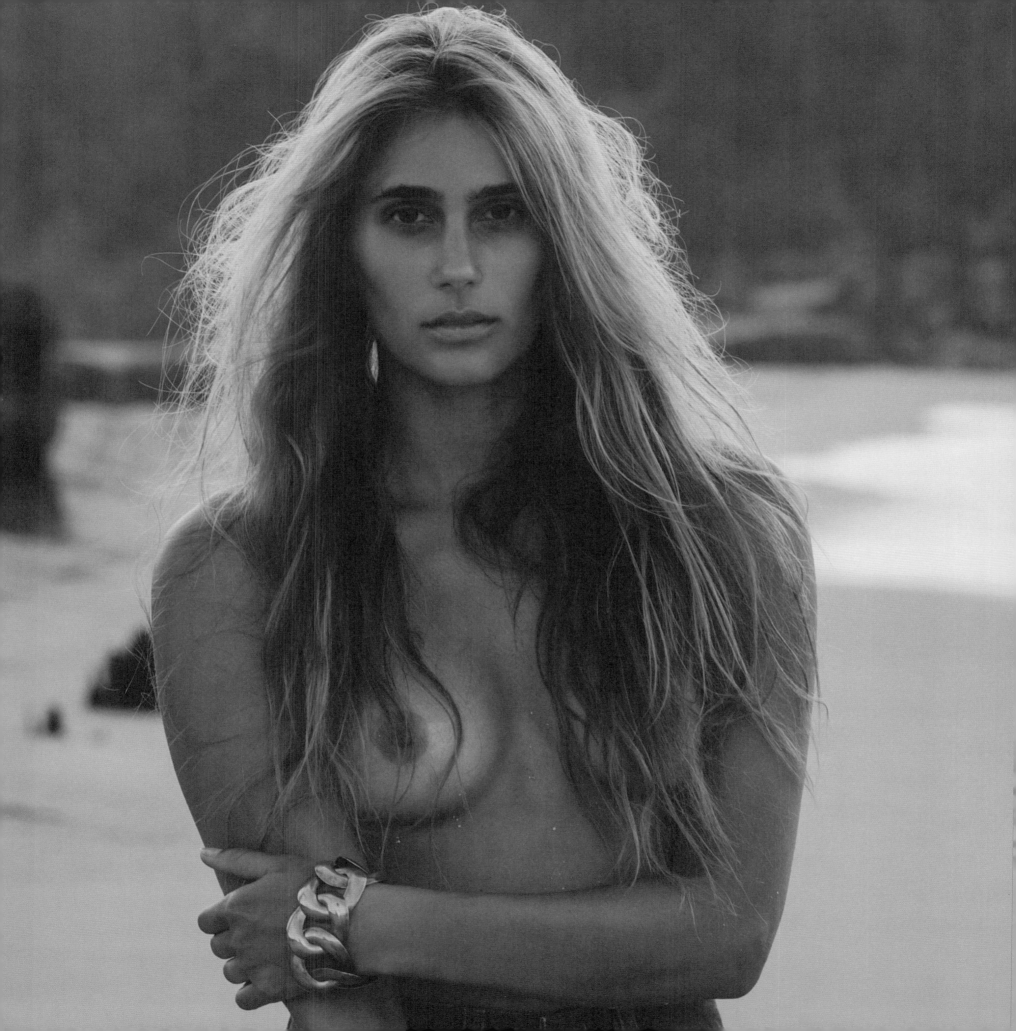

"For me, the most effective way
to find peace in any given moment is
to connect, align, and embody
my Spirit. I start by
grounding in my body
and activating my breath through
activities like yoga and surfing.
And then I open my heart and invite
my spirit in so we can glide through
life together, embodied
on our authentic path.
This guidance and
support keep me living my truth
and that brings me peace."

Perri Ricci
*Mermaid, mom, model, surfer, yogi and
founder of The Puka Project*

"Ride hard with your head up, even in the most difficult times. For what lies ahead is exciting and can't be missed."

Elizabeth Goodwin Welborn
Mom, international polo player, entrepreneur and founder of Stick & Ball

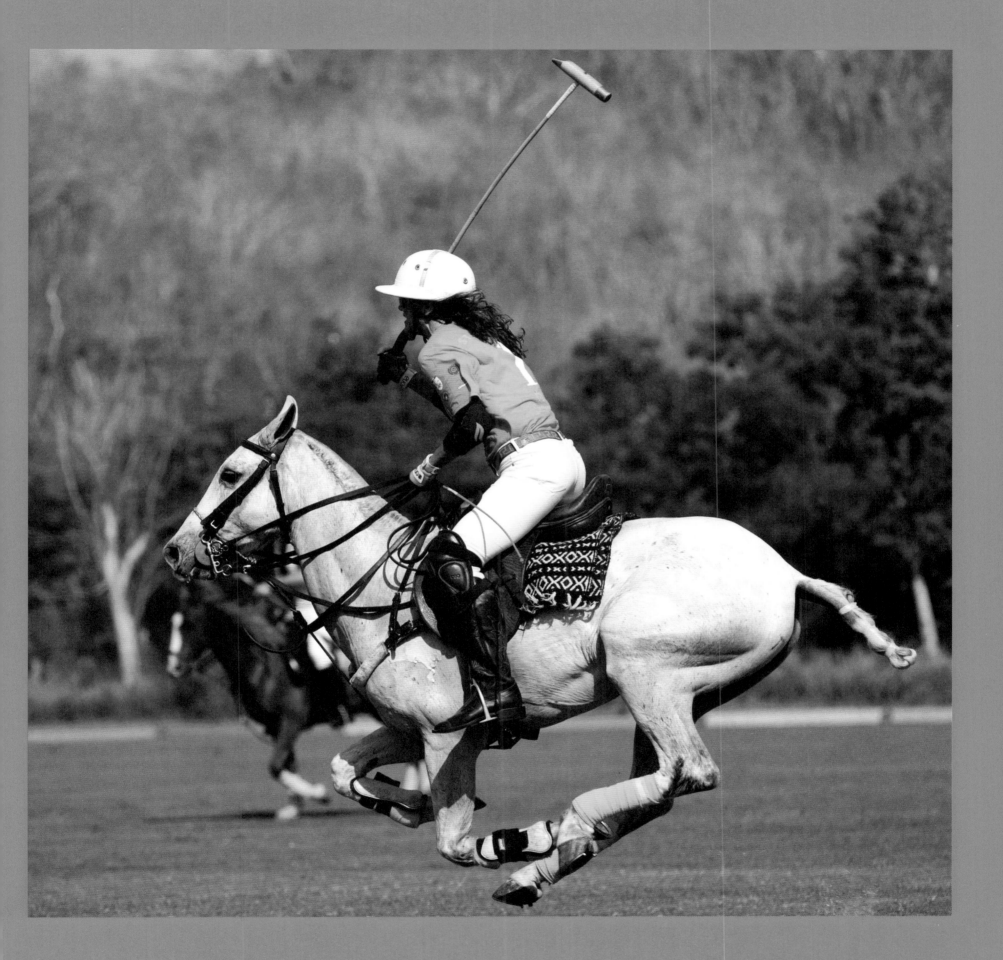

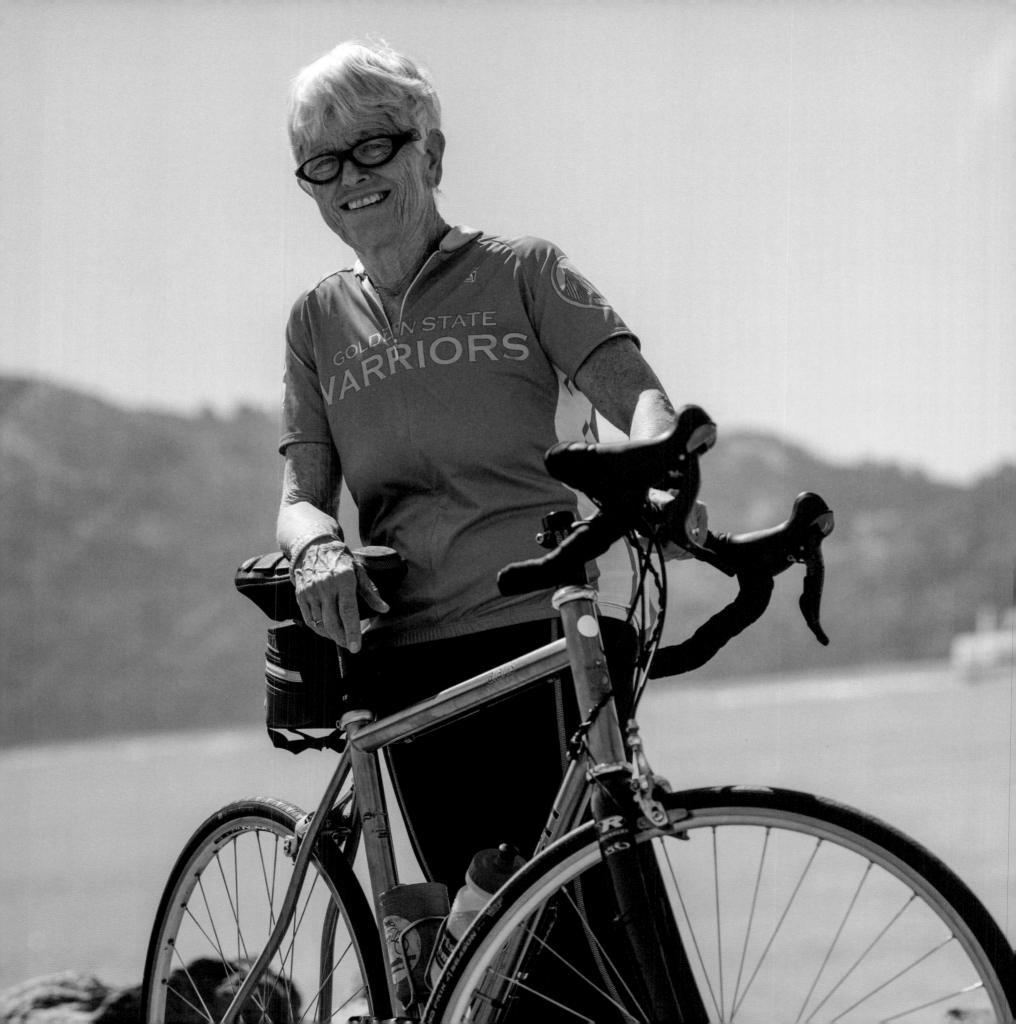

'One of the hardest things to get used to as I age, is that I become more and more invisible. There was a time when every male rider that went past me, would chat me up. Not anymore!"

Agatha Hoff
Mom, grandmother, court commissioner and cyclist

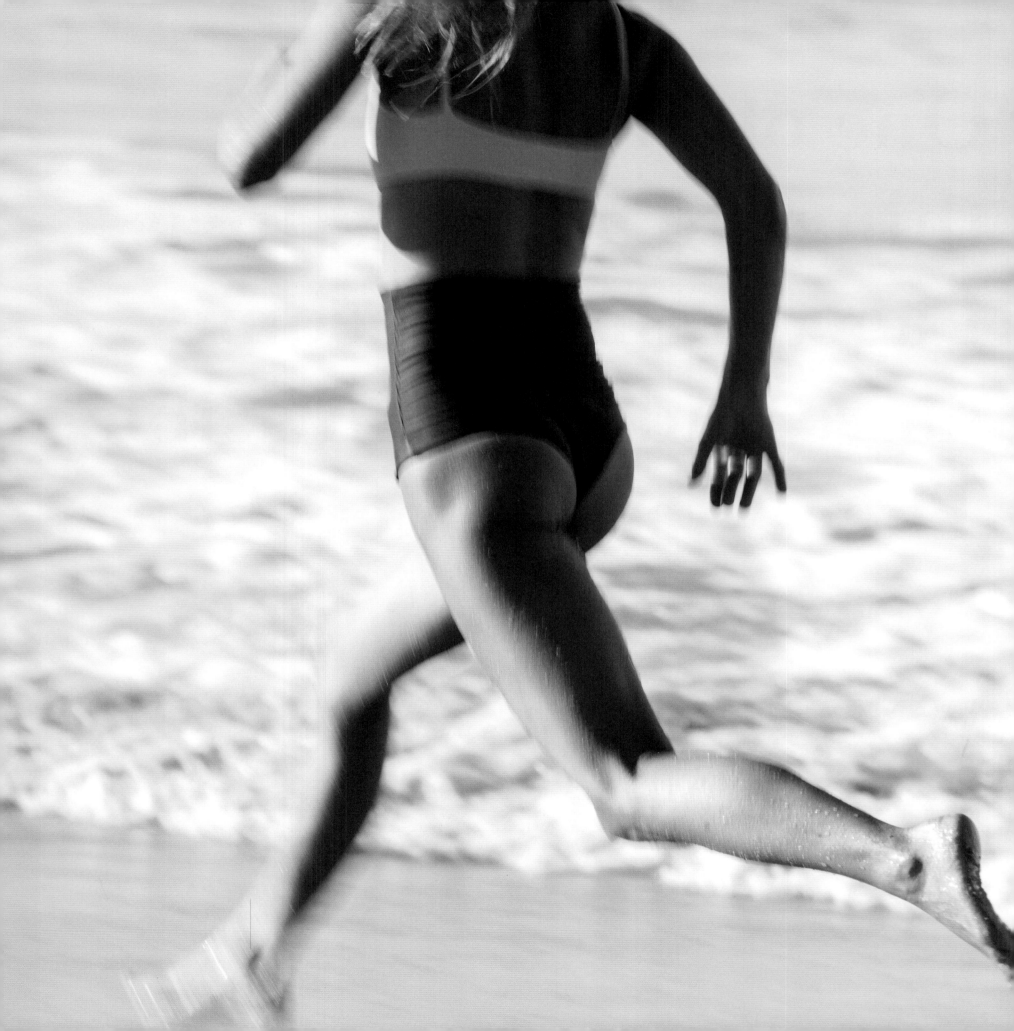

Chapter 15

HOW EXERCISE CONTRIBUTES TO TRUE HEALTH

One of the reasons I wrote this book was to outline the difference between being "healthy" versus being "physically fit". I was working out a ton as a college athlete, yet I was tired and depleted. In this chapter, I talk about how exercise fits into true health and outline how much and what types of exercise you should be doing to achieve a healthy body and mind.

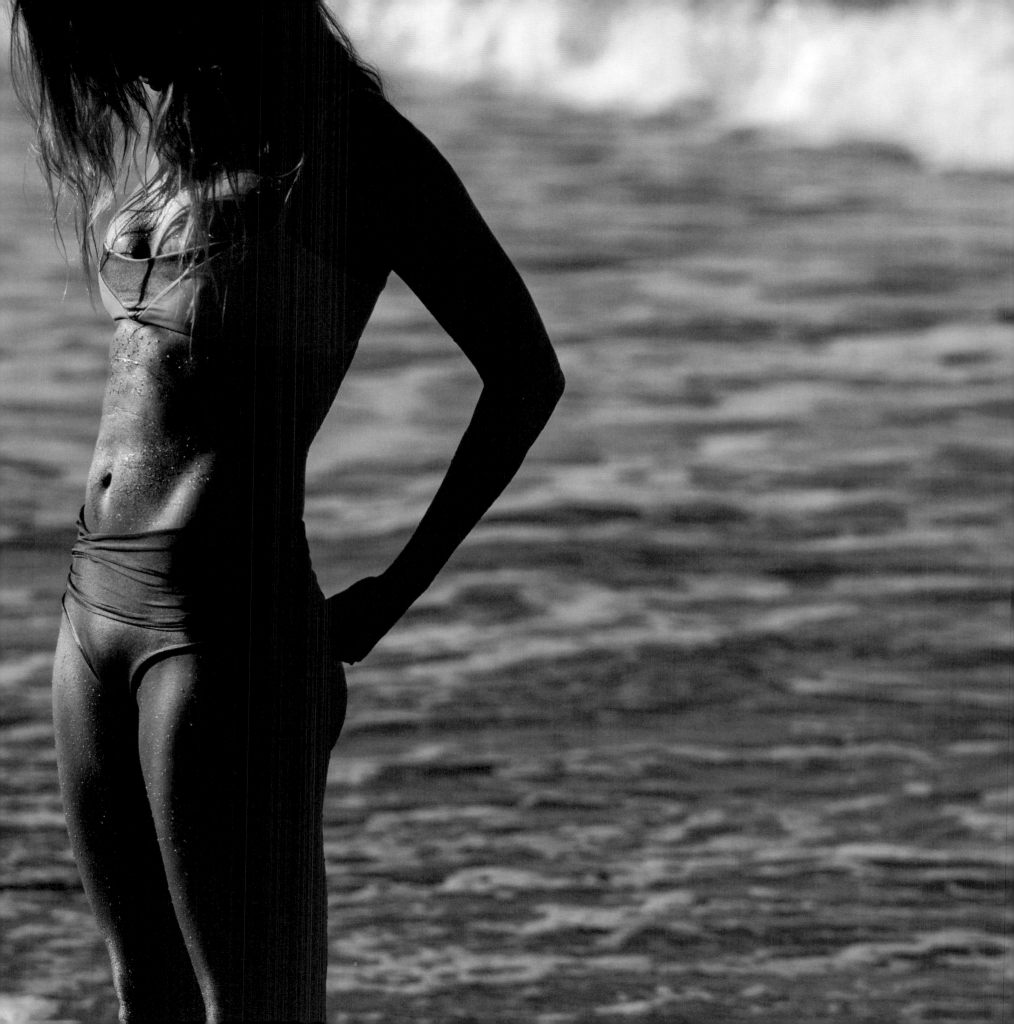

WHY EXERCISE?

We all know that exercise is important. Not only does regular exercise help ward off a range of health conditions – such as stroke, diabetes and many types of cancer — it also acts as a natural antidepressant by stimulating certain brain chemicals, that can leave you happier and more relaxed. Exercise helps you get better, deeper sleep and can put the pizazz back into your sex life.

HOW MUCH EXERCISE DO YOU REALLY NEED?

There is no right formula for how many days or hours per week you should exercise. As a general guideline, you should aim for 30 to 45 minutes of moderate-intensity cardio four to five days a week, as well as weight training to maintain lean body mass and preserve your muscles. Three to five days of weight training for each muscle group, with two to three sets of 12 to 15 repetitions is a good goal, according to personal trainer and fitness expert, Suzie Cooney of Suzie Trains Maui.[37] On the flip side, too much exercise can do more harm than good. "There is that certain type of person who trains intensely and increases their training too much, too fast," says Elizabeth Matzkin, M.D., an assistant professor of orthopedic surgery at Harvard who has seen an increase in rotator cuff and labral tears, sprained ankles, and stress fractures. "Bones are living tissue and if you introduce stress too quickly, then you get hurt."[38]

Like everything, having a balanced workout that includes days of rest is important. Your body needs time off to repair itself, adapt to new strength gains, and avoid overuse injuries. If you become too tired and cannot recover as well, or if your training becomes sloppy and flat, it is time to rest and review.

"The most important sign to really listen to is continual discomfort when you are exercising," explains Claudette Lajam, M.D., assistant professor of orthopedic surgery at NYU Langone Medical Center. "Your body makes pain for a reason, so you need to stop what you are doing if you are feeling it." [39]

WHAT KIND OF EXERCISE SHOULD YOU DO?

As a former competitive athlete, I know the key to working out and staying fit is to find an exercise you like and are excited to do on a regular basis. After a long tennis career, I started surfing eight years ago and quickly fell in love with the sport. It's a hard workout, paddling like crazy to catch the next wave, but it also helps me relax and let go of my worries. Every time I get out of the water, I have a huge smile on my face and I feel great inside and out – being in the water is my own form of personal meditation!

My ideal workout is to do The Dailey Method "barre class", which features elements of Pilates, ballet and yoga, with swimming, cycling (indoor and outdoors) or surfing on the other days. I also do 45 minutes of fast weight training twice a week and rest on Sundays. I don't time my swimming or surfing, but instead let the ocean (and my body) tell me when I have had enough.

Here is some additional exercise advice from the experts:

Train outdoors: Suzie Cooney, Suzie Trains Maui. Training outdoors is really a great way to enjoy all that nature can bring – from beach training to trail running, to surfing, stand-up paddle boarding and swimming, it never gets boring. You can easily incorporate core exercises, balance and strength training by doing walking lunges, climbing up a sand dune or hill and sprinting or swimming at the very end of your workout. Even walking in waist deep water is great for the legs. Working out with a group of friends is a great way to catch up and enjoy every bit of this work out time together. On Maui, I use coconuts and coral as markers for agility work, core planks and then use resistance bands to add for upper body strength training. Then we may run down the beach along the water's edge, followed by a few uphill sand dune runs. As our reward, we swim and cool down in the natural reef pool.

Alternate aerobic training with resistance work: Tom Rosencrantz, USA Cycling Coach. Weekly workouts that combine aerobic activity (such as biking and running) with two days of resistance work/core strength and functional training are best. But working on machines at a gym for resistance training is a great way to keep the muscles toned, strong and balanced.

Strengthen your core and quiet your mind: Jill Dailey, The Dailey Method. I recommend exercise that simultaneously strengthens your core, stretches your body and quiets your mind. There is yoga, Pilates and, my favorite, barre work. Jill Dailey's motto is to "align your body, mind and spirit", which is a key and integral part of being nourished from the inside out. The Dailey Method classes are an ever-evolving mix of micro-movements that tone, elongate and isolate the muscles. Engaging the core helps align the body, stabilize the muscles closest to the spine and improve spinal health, which is critical as we age.

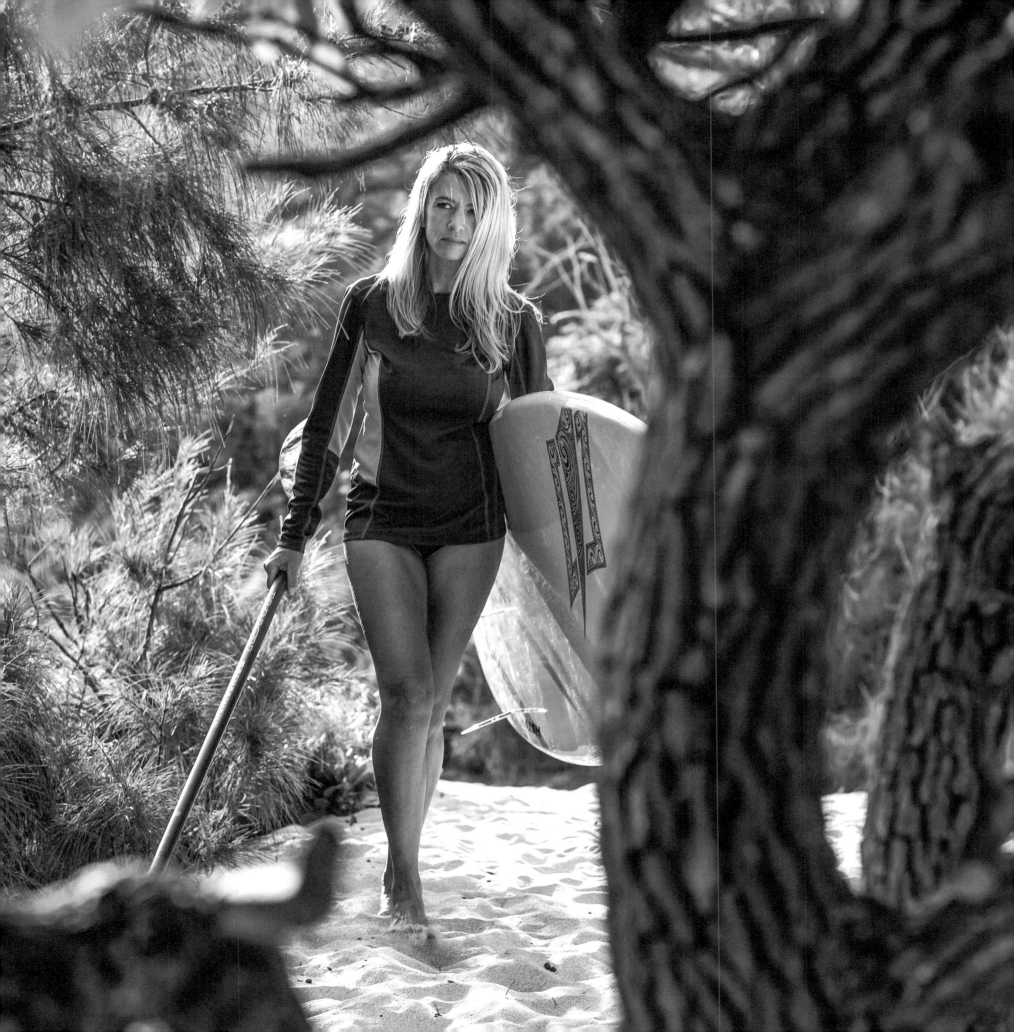

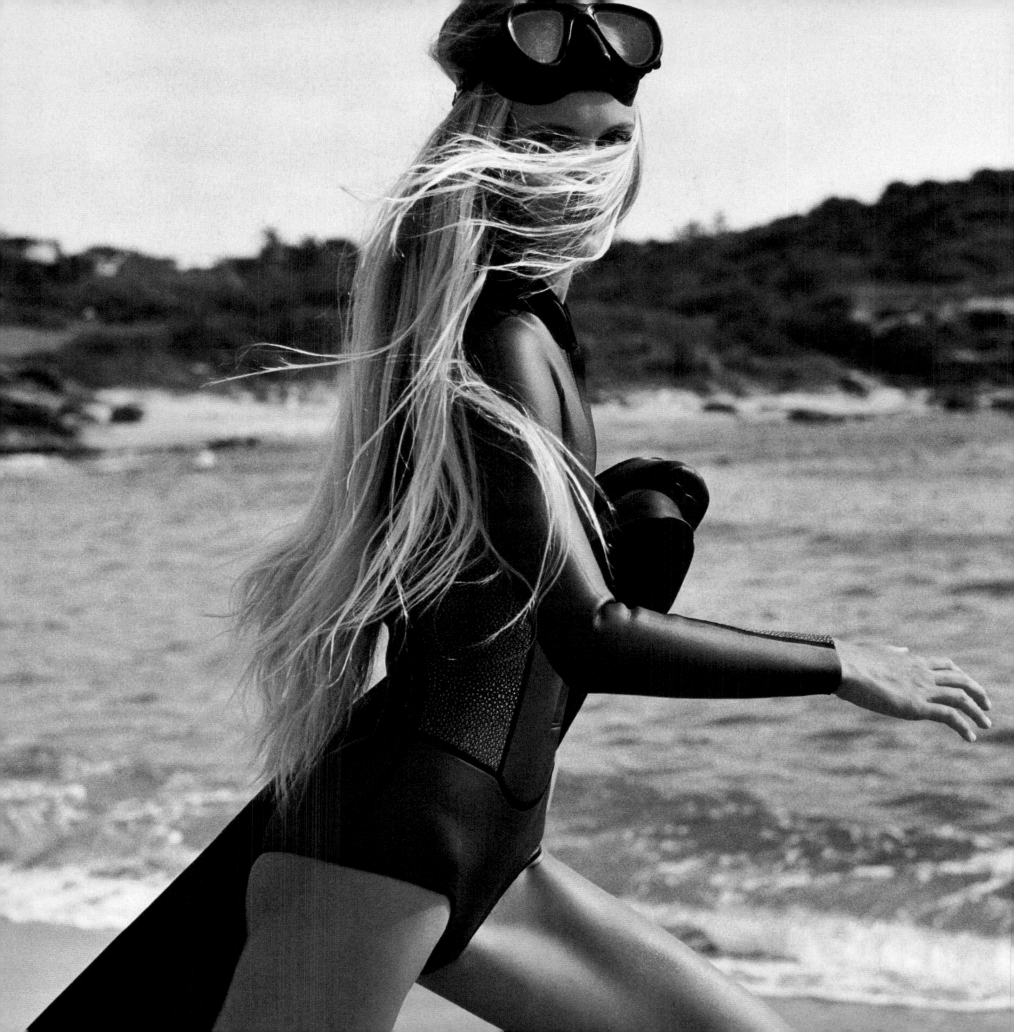

Chapter 16

WEEKLY SAMPLE WORKOUTS FROM TOP ATHLETES

Here I outline three effective exercise routines from top trainers and athletes that you can build into your schedule.

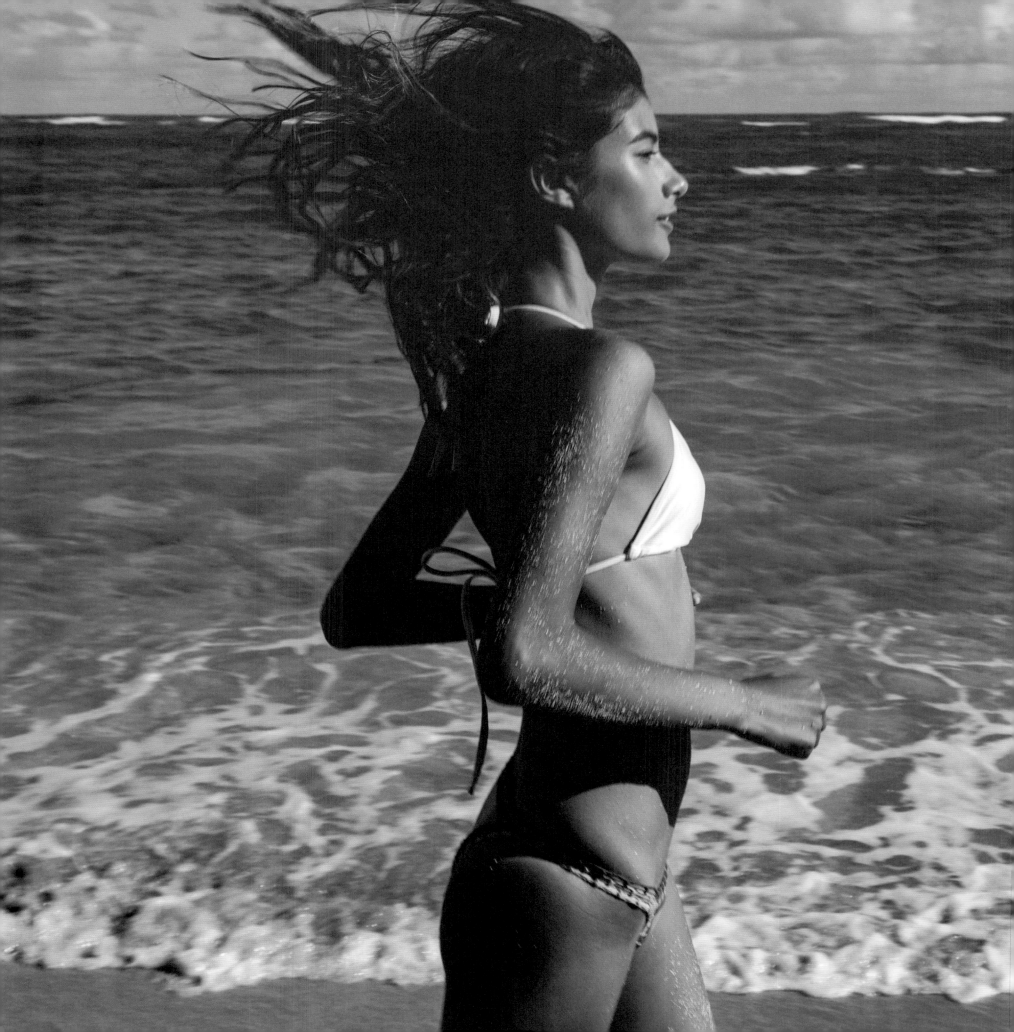

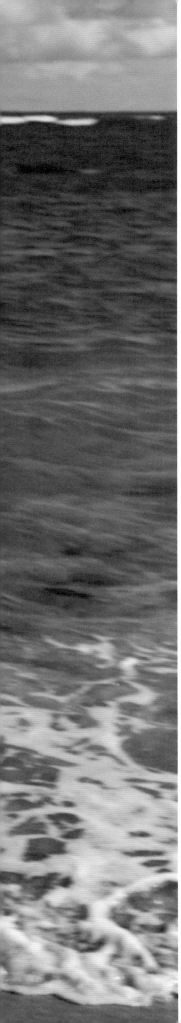

INDOOR (GYM)/OUTDOOR WORKOUT
Sandra Holbrook James, Competitive Triathlete, Health Coach

Monday: Swim 30 minutes
- Warm-up for 10 minutes alternating using pull buoy and kick board
- 4 x 50m alternating sets with 25 non-freestyle stroke and 25 freestyle stroke
- 4 x 100m with a 10-second rest in between sets
- Cool down alternating using pool buoy and kick board

Tuesday: Bike 45-60 minutes
- Mix flat and hilly terrain
- Maximum effort when climb to elevate heart rate

Wednesday: Strength/core 45–60 minutes
- Quick 5 to 10-minute warm up on jump rope or treadmill
- Alternate dynamic movements with bands, Bosu ball or sand bags

Thursday: Run 45 minutes
- Warm-up 15 minutes
- 20-minute tempo pace (steady pace with effort but not uncomfortable)
- Cool down (10 minutes)

Friday: Rest or yoga

Saturday: Run or bike 60 minutes
- All aerobic

Sunday: Yoga

Duration can vary as well as intensity based on your fitness. Always include a warm-up and cool down. Depending on where you live in the world you can choose any of the following: cross-country skiing, skate skiing, snow shoeing, downhill skiing or running (inside or outside) and yoga.

WINTER WORKOUT
Sandra Holbrook James, Competitive Triathlete, Health Coach

Monday: Skate ski or classic ski or outdoor run 1 hour
- Warm-up for 15 minutes
- 30-minute tempo pace with some effort
- Cool down for 15 minutes

Tuesday: 45-minute run or snowshoe with option of skate/classic skiing

Wednesday: Yoga or rest

Thursday: Downhill ski all day or classic ski

Friday: 1 hour aerobic snow shoe
- Include hills

Saturday: Skate/classic ski or run 1 hour
- Include all terrain and mixed tempos

Sunday: Yoga/Rest

'BALLET BARRE' WORKOUT
The DAILEY METHOD by Jill Dailey, BARRE, PILATES and YOGA

Below is a sample Dailey Method Barre Class schedule for one week, which I love. I certainly see results.[40]

Monday: Daily Barre Class (appropriate for all levels of students). Quick and steady pace, core training, targeted leg strengthening, various planks, arm work with free weights and full body stretching. Great upbeat music for one hour. Focus is on priority positioning and movement is layered on after form and alignment.

Tuesday: Dailey Interval Class (a fast-paced, 45 minute class that combines periods of high- and low-intensity movement for optimal cardiovascular results). The heart rate is elevated and brought down throughout the class, while recovery periods remain active. The interval training and fun, upbeat music give you the power and energy to bring your best to the more intense portions of The Dailey Barre.

Wednesday: Dailey Barre Class

Thursday: Dailey Fusion Class (a faster paced one-hour class that fuses the alignment focused elements of barre with the intensity of interval to give your full body strength and stretching experience with intermittent blasts of cardiovascular fun). A challenging workout that will guide you towards deepening your practice at a more energetic pace. This class is not recommended for first-time students.

Friday: Dailey Barre Class

Saturday: Speedwalking or hiking with effort

Sunday: Rest

This way you get two days of cardiovascular exercise and three days of strength and toning that works best for your body. If you are lucky enough to have a Dailey Cycle near you or you love cardio then do two Dailey Barre and three Dailey classes of your choice. "We are all different and need to listen to our bodies and also enjoy our workouts," says Jill Dailey.

Alternatively, on Monday, Wednesday, Friday you could choose to substitute any yoga or Pilates classes instead of barre, and on Tuesday and Thursday you could substitute with a 45 minute run or one hour fast-paced hike.
To find a studio nearest you go to *thedaileymethod.com*.

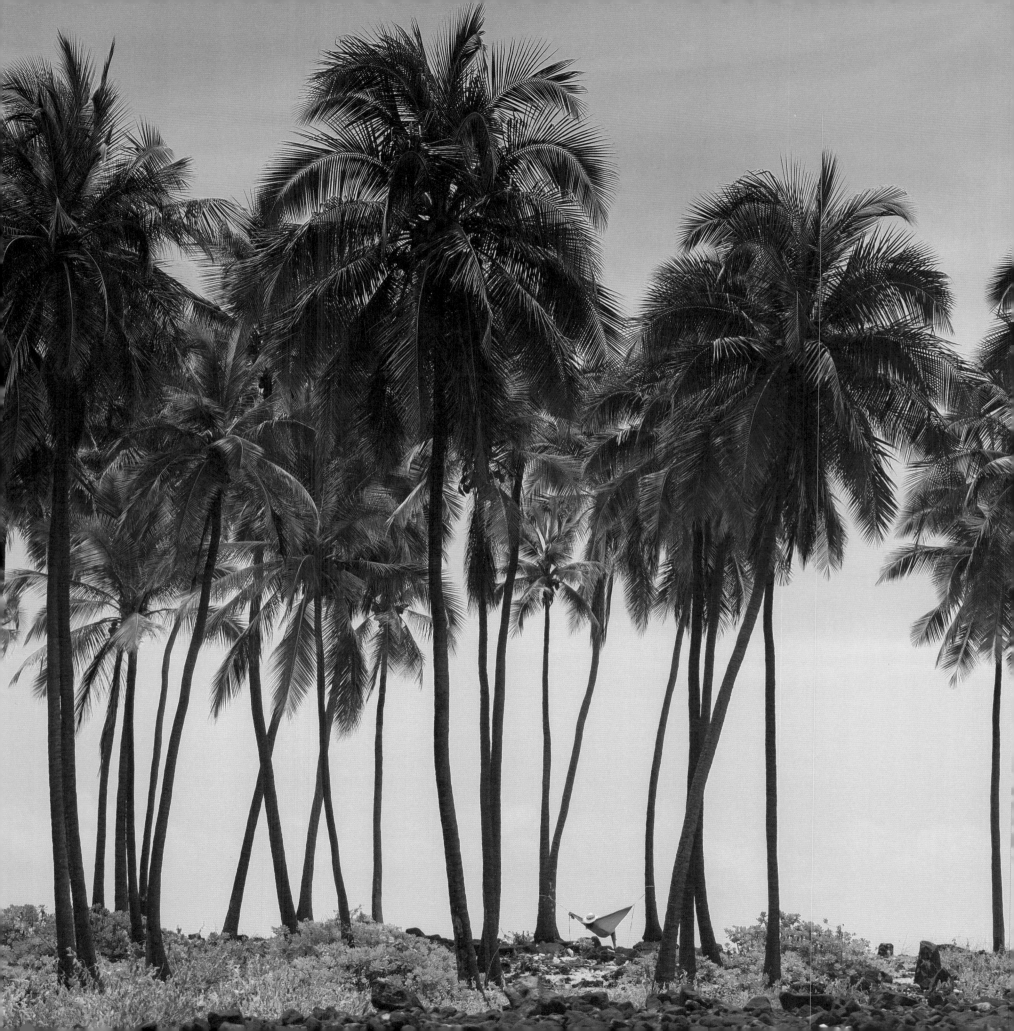

Chapter 17

SLEEP

Restful sleep is the foundation of your mental and physical well being. I learned this the hard way a few years ago when I suffered a three-month period of insomnia. I was ready to check myself into a hospital. Part of the cause, I realized later on, was the stress and anxiety I was experiencing in my marriage. I was not dealing with my emotional imbalance, and it was getting the best of me.

I was on vacation in Maui when I decided to try meditating. I searched the Internet for beginning meditations and found some calming music and mantras to follow. That night, I slept better than I had in years. I started meditating for 30 minutes twice a day, every day. Slowly, my sleep got back on track, and other things changed for the better, too. My skin improved, my appetite increased, as did my energy and focus. I felt like a human again, and my kids had their "real" mother back!

Sleep is when your body and muscles repair themselves; they build protein, release growth hormones and create new tissue. Lack of sleep can lead to a host of health issues, including obesity, diabetes, immune problems and increased risk of cancer. Plus, it raises your risk of accidents and occupational errors.[41]

Most people need at least six to eight hours of sleep a night. To get a good night's sleep, you should make sure your bedtime is consistent so your body can get into a rhythm. You should also empty your bedroom of electronics. Our devices, including iPhones, laptops and televisions, emit a blue light that has been found to interfere with melatonin production. Melatonin is one of the hormones responsible for our sleep cycles. It encourages our peaceful rest and reaches its peak between 2am and 4am, gradually ebbing so that we can rise in the morning.[42] The blue light from electronics decreases melatonin production and interrupts your sleep cycle.

TIPS FOR GETTING A GOOD NIGHT'S SLEEP
- Eat a light and early dinner.
- No intensive activities or exercise after 8pm.
- Take a calming warm 10 to 15 minute bath or shower (after, slather and massage your entire body with a calming moisturizing oil. I like pure raw coconut oil with a lemongrass or lavender essential oil).
- Drink a small cup of warm herbal tea.
- To clear your mind of your busy day, try journaling.
- No electronics in your bed or bedroom. You may read but nothing too heavy.
- Once you are in bed, turn off all lights. Close your eyes and focus on relieving any tensions you might have. Just simply let go and relax.

Note: If you still have trouble falling asleep, try meditating to calm your mind. You can find meditations online at *chopra.com, or see more guided meditations listed on page 241.*

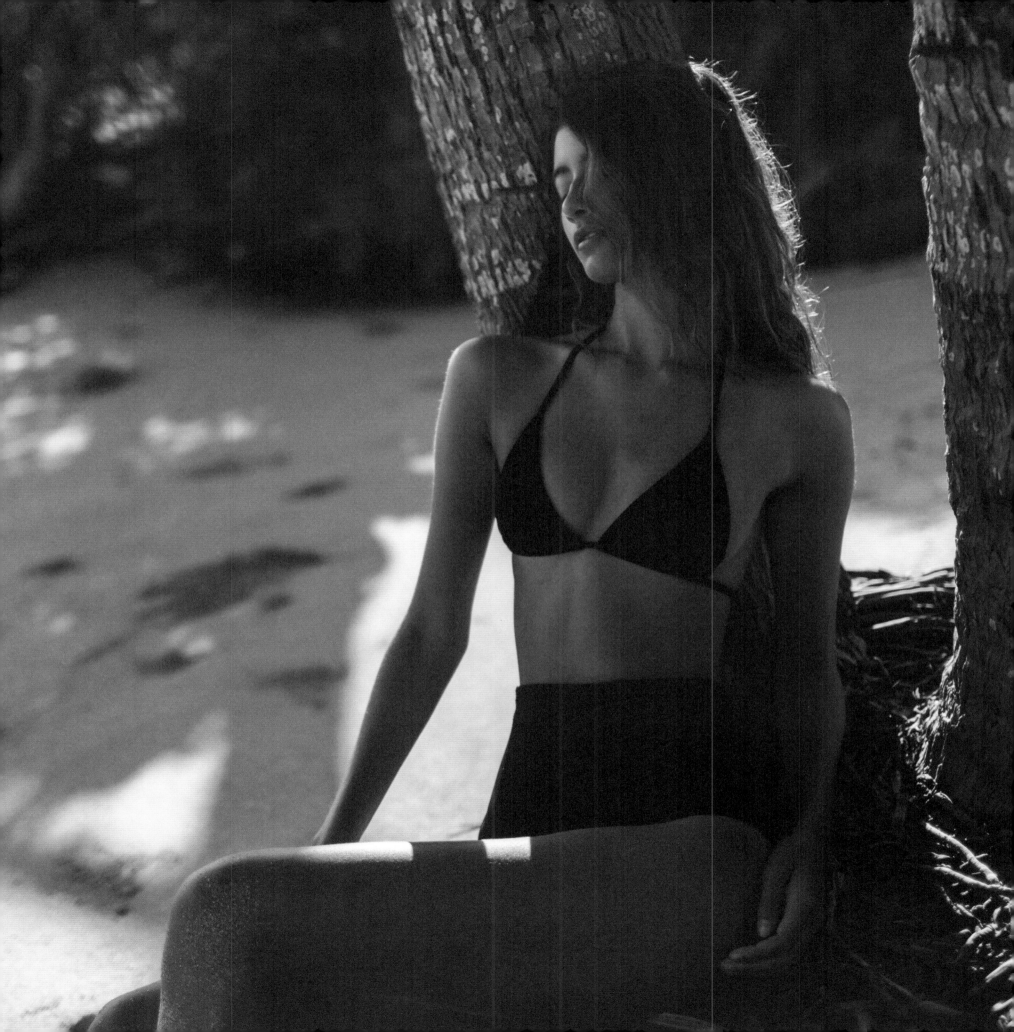

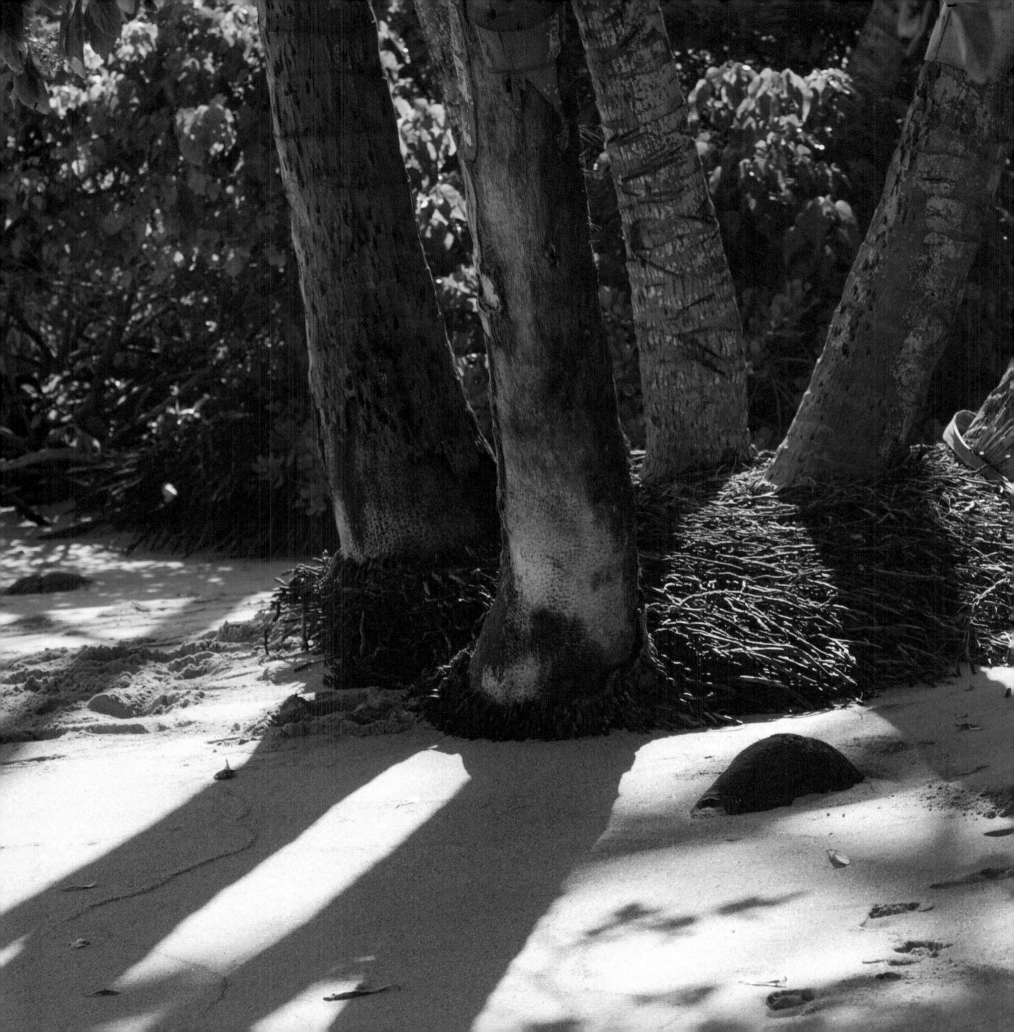

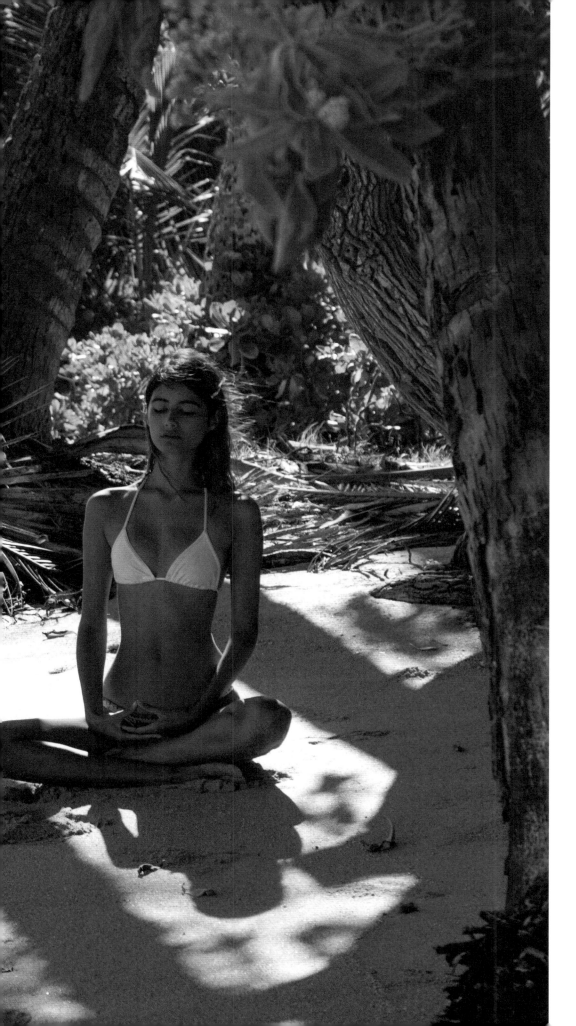

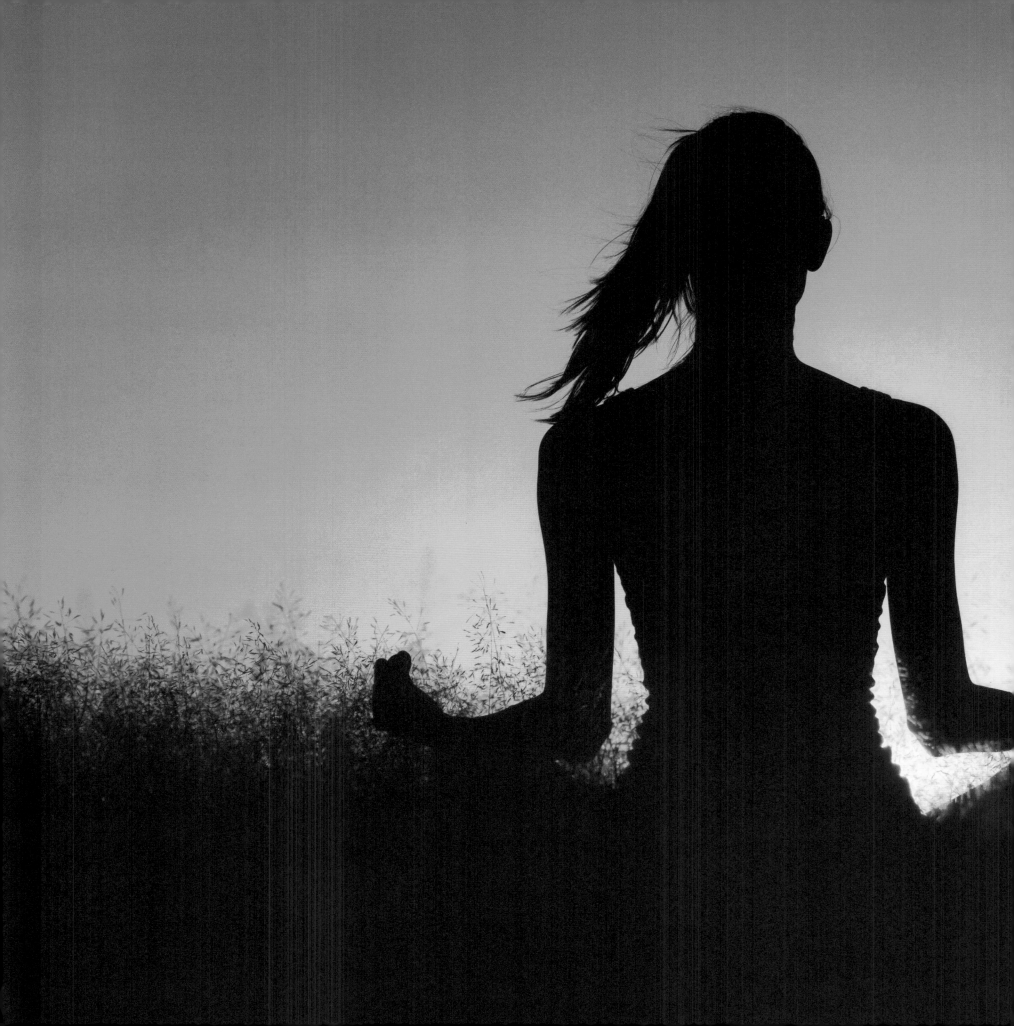

Chapter 18

THE HEALING POWER OF MEDITATION

What I realized and finally learned at the age of 40, is that it takes everything combined in life – it's not just about one thing. This is what I have experienced and I'm currently writing about: in order to truly be well you have to have all of the components working together. It's the same as a spider web. You pull one thread out of the web and the web will collapse. I am learning that I need to really manage my stress and make it a ritual that I work on every day. It is different for everyone, but working on many parts of this intricate web, including daily meditation, is a formula that works and can be used by all.

We spend most of our lives looking outward to the world, believing that the source of happiness is external to ourselves. But it isn't. True happiness comes from within, and meditation helps us access it.

I used to think of surfing as my own personal form of meditation. Being alone on the waves, feeling the water in my hair, the repetition of paddling out and sailing along on the top of a wave – it would quiet my mind and wipe out any thoughts or concerns about work, family or marital stress. Yet, despite the peace I felt when I surfed (or went for a long run), I did not understand the benefits of true meditation until I went on a six-day retreat at the Deepak Chopra Center in Southern California.

During this retreat, we did a guided meditation with an instructor twice a day – once in the morning at 7am and again at 6:30 pm. We would start with two to three deep breaths, eyes closed and begin with the guided question, "Who am I?" We were each given a mantra that was decided by our date of birth and time we were born. We would repeat this mantra over and over until it seemed to somehow disappear into thin air. After 30 minutes, I would feel relaxed and my mind was surprisingly clear.

The key to mastering any type of meditation practice is to do it every day. Start with shorter sessions if you need, but the goal is to work up to 30 minutes twice a day. This is when you truly see healing and a clear focus beginning to form.

ACCORDING TO *CHOPRA.COM*:
According to Deepak Chopra, meditation is not about forcing your mind to be quiet; rather it's a process to "rediscover the quietness that's already there".[43]

Behind the screen of our internal dialogue is the silence of pure awareness – a silence that is not disturbed by thoughts of the past or concerns of the future. The actual silence we experience in meditation is the "gap" between thoughts. Experiencing this path of calmness or quiet zone, expanded awareness allows you to recognize that your essential self is not the ongoing traffic of thoughts that fill your mind, but the silent witness to your thoughts, words and actions. Daily practice of meditation helps establish inner quietness in your everyday life, providing greater access to creativity and enabling you to make life-affirming choices.[44]

My mediation practice has become a way of life for me and has begun to live inside my body and mind, so that even when I'm not actively meditating, I am still reaping the benefits. I feel as if nothing can hurt me now – no bad words thrown my way or terrible anxiety and stress can make it through my body. Meditation also brings a feeling of open compassion and wellness for the world. I feel like I am on top of a tree branch looking down at millions of smaller trees on the Earth that need help in some indirect way. The trees (or humans) all look ruffled from the numerous storms of stress that blow in and out each day. They look lost, tired, stressed and some even angry. Meditation helps get us back to the core or root of who we really are. It brings us back to the simplest, purest form of human life.

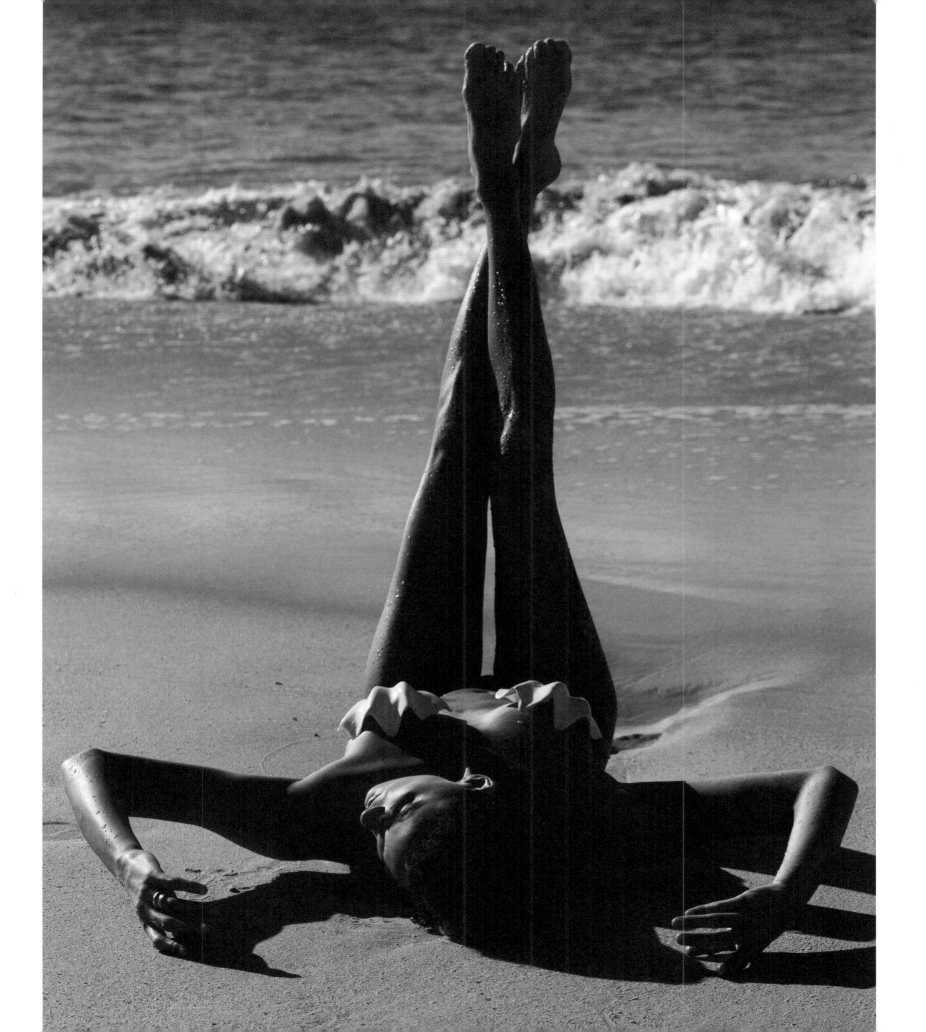

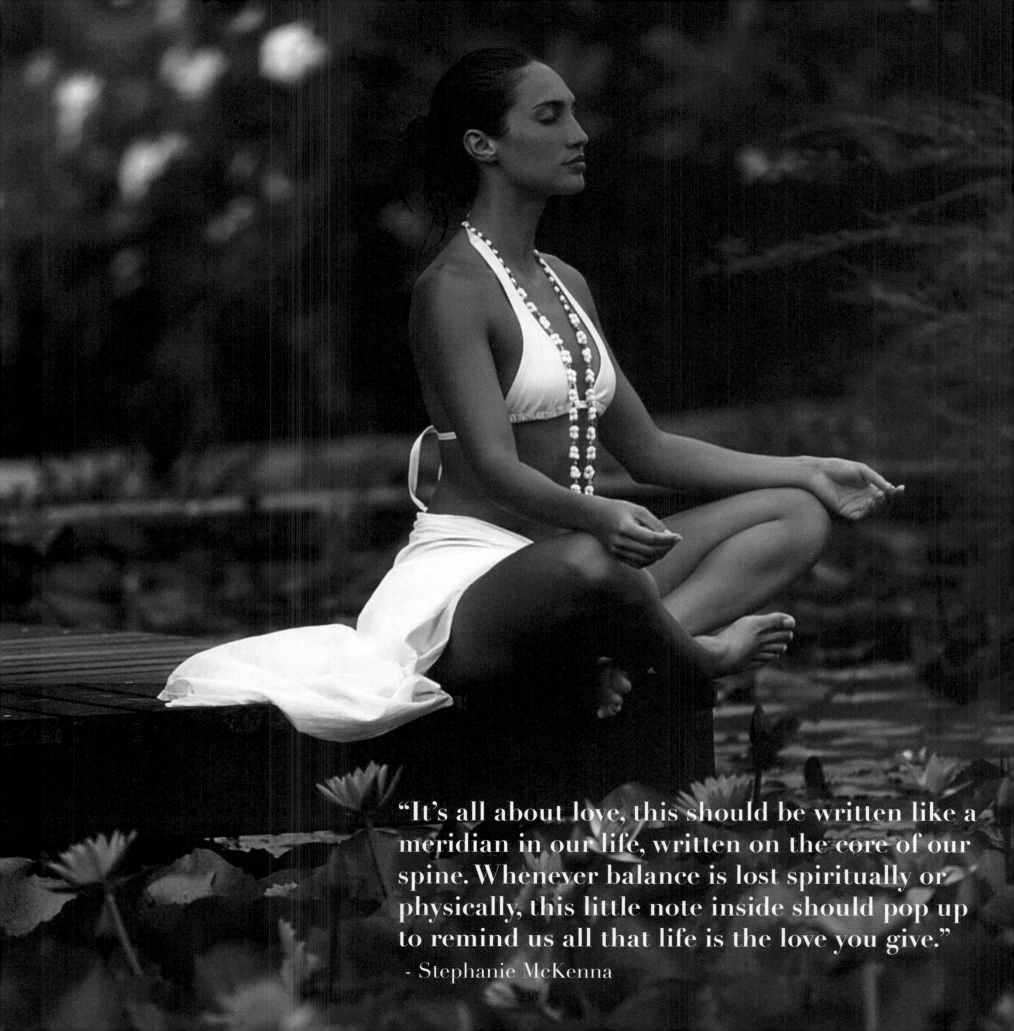

"It's all about love, this should be written like a meridian in our life, written on the core of our spine. Whenever balance is lost spiritually or physically, this little note inside should pop up to remind us all that life is the love you give."
- Stephanie McKenna

Chapter 19

SIMPLE GUIDELINES
FOR MEDITATION

It's important to start with a good understanding of the

basic principles of meditation. While there are no hard and fast rules,

there are guidelines that can help you learn how to begin.

You can adapt these guidelines to your lifestyle and schedule.

MEDITATION GUIDELINES

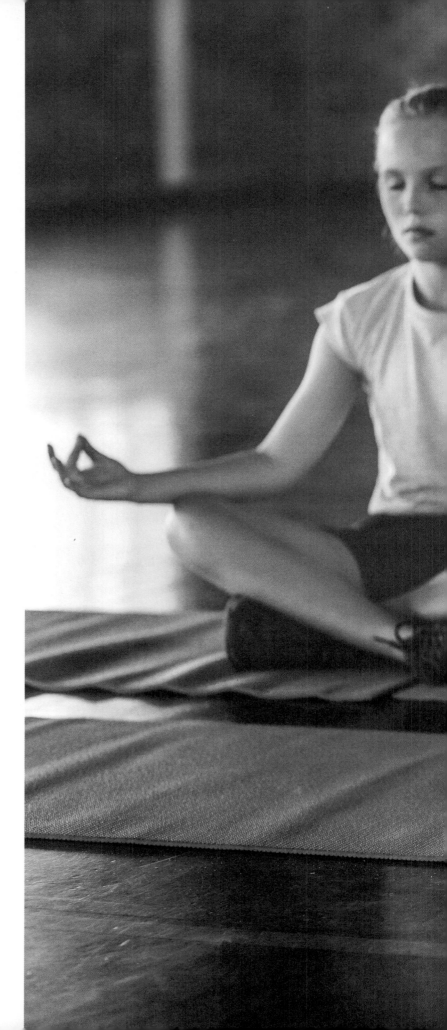

- Your mantra is used for its sound or vibration quality. Let go of any association that attaches any meaning to your mantra. It will hold you on the level of the mind and slow your entry into the gap. Your mantra can be figured out by your birth date and time you were born.

- Meditate sitting up. Lying down is associated with going to sleep and is not recommended. Sit up in whatever position is comfortable so your attention is not being continually drawn to sensations in your body.

- Always close your eyes to meditate. When your eyes are open, our attention usually wanders all over the place, which is opposite to the inward process of meditation.

- Whenever possible, meditate in an environment free of disturbances. Remember, that you can actually meditate anywhere you can sit down and close your eyes.

- For maximum benefits, I recommend meditating twice a day for up to 30 minutes each time, depending on your age. The best times to meditate are first thing in the morning before breakfast or early evening before dinner. Meditation usually makes the mind more alert and energetic, so it's generally recommended not to meditate before bedtime. Consistency of meditation is very important, so do what you can each day.

- From time to time, you may become distracted by the thoughts in your mind, or saying your mantra wrong, too fast, jumbled or too slow, or outside noises in the environment. This is a normal part of the process, so don't beat yourself up. However, anytime during your meditation that you realize you are not thinking your mantra, just return right back to it.

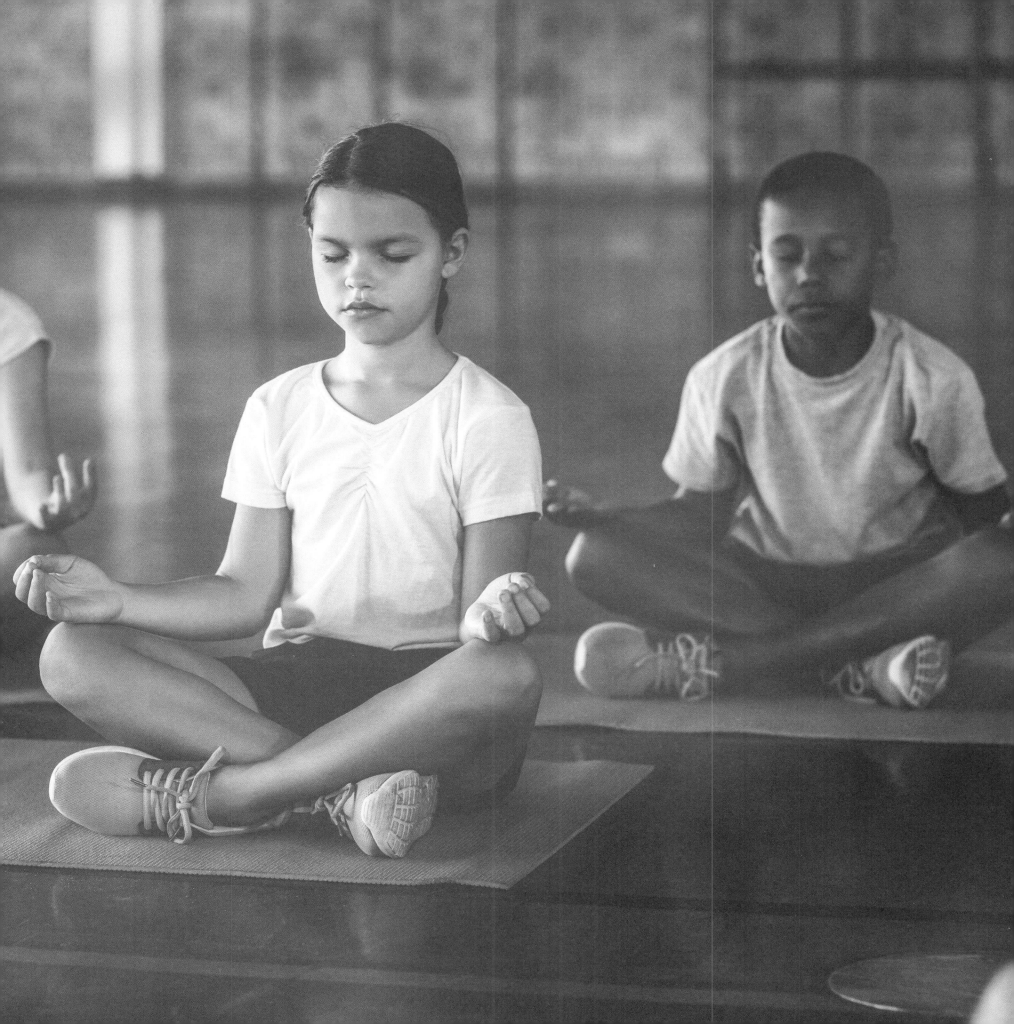

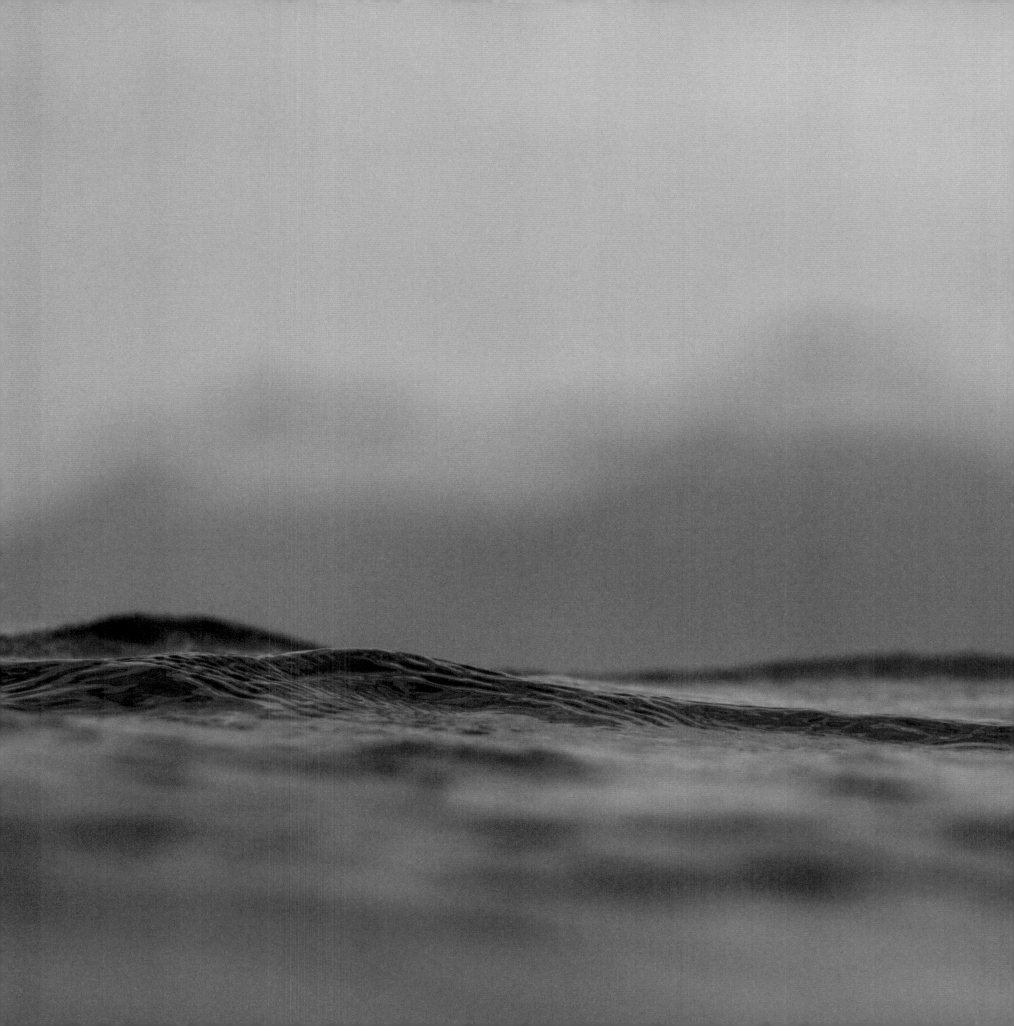

Chapter 20

GUIDED ONLINE MEDITATION PRACTICES

Here are a few recommended apps and tools

to guide you in your meditation.

BUDDHIFY is for those of us who are busy and on the go. This app gives mindfulness a modern twist.

HEADSPACE is great for beginning meditators and was created by a Buddhist monk. This app requires that you first complete a 10 day introductory meditation program and then you can access the other programs.

CALM helps you de-stress from a busy day. I love that you can customize the background scenery and noise to make your meditation a virtual retreat.

WHIL was created by the founders of Lululemon, and guides you through traditional meditation practices. You can also choose yoga programs – depending on your mood, intention and time, you can choose from a database of numerous options that will suit you.

INSIGHT TIMER is for master meditators. This allows you to can choose a soft background noise, time and alarm to finish your session.

CHOPRA is a great resource for guided meditation practices, and offers continuing courses throughout the year – each with a unique theme. Meditation sessions go from five minutes to an hour; I often use this site because it's fast, free and easy to get started.

SIMPLE HABIT is designed by a Harvard psychologist. These five-minute meditations focus on topics such as reducing stress, improving sleep, boosting focus and memory, and preparing for difficult conversations or talks.

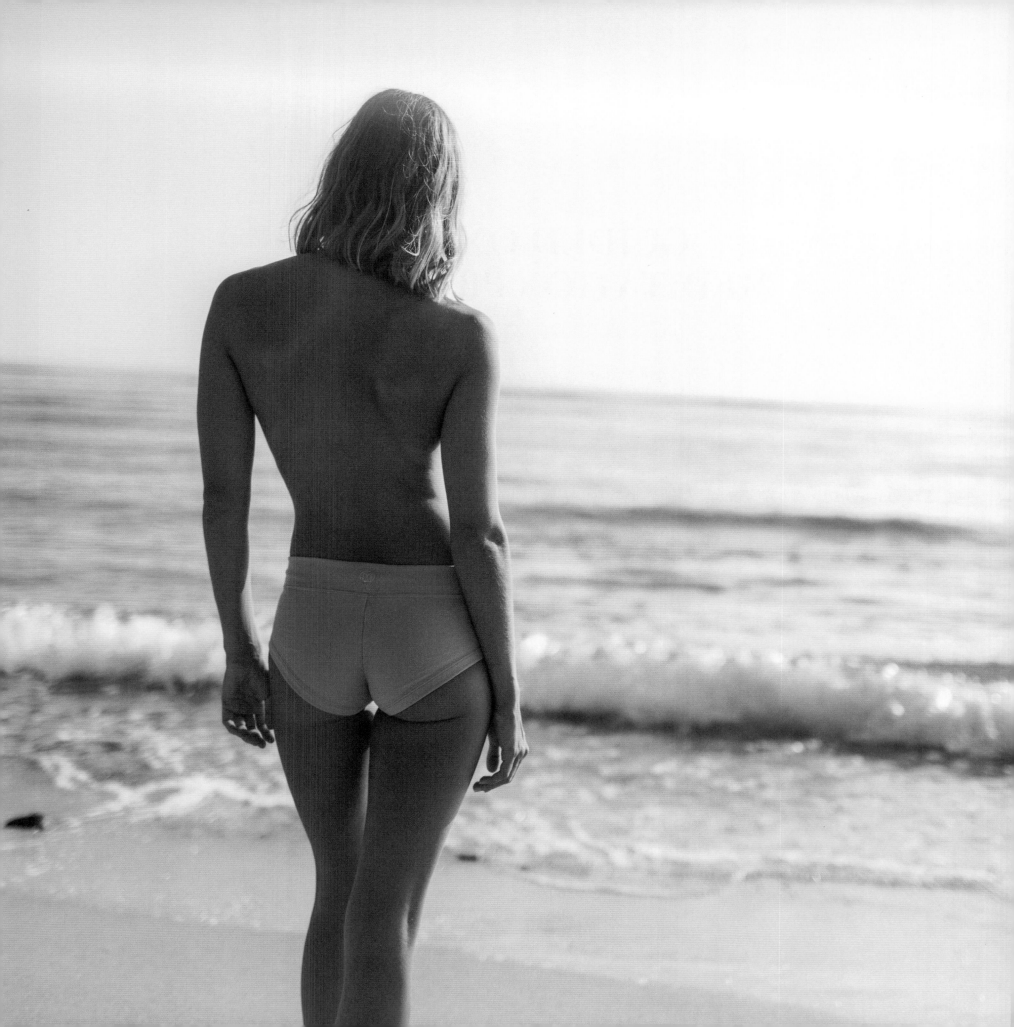

Chapter 21

THE HEALING POWER OF TOUCH

Research has proven the healing power of human touch. In one landmark study, 16

married women were subjected to the threat of a mild electric shock; touching their

husbands' hands brought immediate relief from the resulting anxiety. [45]

Even a stranger's touch was somewhat calming.

"We know that anxiety decreases immune function and makes

you get sick more often," says study author Jim Coan, Ph.D.,

a neuroscientist at the University of Virginia.

"If touch can help you be less anxious, you're more likely to stay well."

MASSAGE THERAPY

Massage therapy can make you more alert and lessen symptoms of depression such as fatigue and irritability, according to the Touch Research Institute at the University of Miami School of Medicine.[46] I learned this first-hand when I attended a wellness seminar at the Chopra Center, which offered both mediation and massage in one package. I was so stressed and filled with anxiety when I arrived at the seminar, but I realized after my first treatment on the first day how powerful and healing the human touch is and what an impact it has on our mind, body and spirit. Here, I share one of the most powerful healing treatments I received at the Chopra Center: Ayurvedic massage.

AYURVEDIC MASSAGE

Ayurveda is an ancient lifestyle practice that aims to create harmony within the body. Practiced widely in India, it is thought that Ayurveda originated more than 400 years ago, making it one of the oldest systems of wellbeing known to mankind. It is based on the philosophy of health and lifestyle that treats the whole person and not just the symptoms. Ayurvedic massage treats the whole body (physically, mentally and emotionally) through touch and the use of essential oils that are chosen to suit your "dosha", or energy. The massage techniques used include tapping, kneading and squeezing as well as the more traditional massage strokes you would expect. The style and flow of the massage is determined by who you are, and what your body needs for balance and wellbeing at the time.[47]

My first Ayurvedic massage treatment started with a series of long massage strokes up and down my entire body. They were incredibly healing, warming and nurturing. Ayurvedic sprays and oils used during the treatment are a big part of the healing process. They open up your senses and help put you in a meditative state.

A separate Ayurvedic massage used circular movements around the joints with amazing long strong strokes up and down the limbs. Hot oil was poured on my head for about 15 minutes and it continually ran into my scalp and all through my head. It was a powerful feeling that melted away all stress and negative emotions. When the oil was on my forehead, it felt like I was floating in the sea. This was all going on with the sounds of ocean waves playing in the background and the smell of the Ayurvedic oils. My massage therapist was tuned in with all the stresses and senses throughout my body, and the treatment washed every bit of stress away.

When I lay there calmly at the end of the treatment, I started to see an emerald green light fill my eyes while they were closed. My therapist told me that this was my chakra showing through. A green chakra is connected to your heart. As my green chakra left, I was already seeing a white light or (white aura color) as my eyes remained closed, which represents peace, balance and harmony.

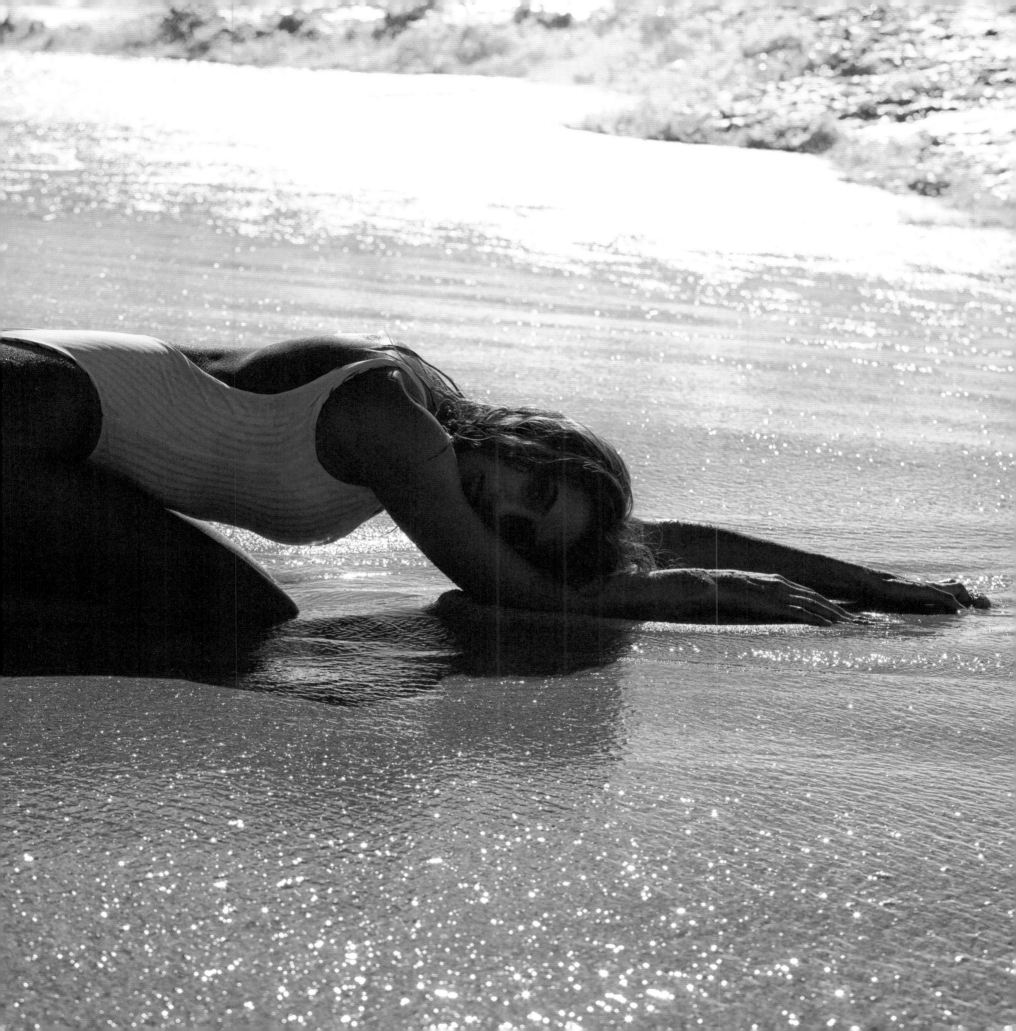

RESOURCES

BLENDERS (HIGH-SPEED)
Blentec – *blentec.com*
Vitamix – *vitamix.com*

INGREDIENTS

OMEGAS
Ahiflower Oil – *amazon.com, epuresolutions.com*

BUSHFOOD AUSTRALIAN SUPERFOODS – *projectyoubewell.com*
Kakadu Plum
Riberry
Davidson Plum
Quandong

MATCHA – *breakawaymatcha.com, kissmeorganics.com*

MILA CHIA SEED – *genesispure.com/alohasusan*
Raw Whole Chia Seeds – *nuts.com*

E3 LIVE BOTANICAL ALGAE – *e3live.com*

GOLDEN SUPERFOODS – *nuts.com*
Goji Berries
Hemp Seed
Maca Powder
Wheatgrass Powder
Mulberries
Cacao Powder
Spirulina
Chlorella
Amla Powder – feelgood.org
Maqui Berry Powder – *feelgood.org*
Sacha Inchi powder – *mrm-usa.com*

CHAI – *us.pranachai.com/collections/shop*

LAVENDER FLOWERS – *feelgood.org*

MEDICINAL MUSHROOMS
6 Mushroom Full Spectrum Extract Blend – *healingspiritfarm.com*
10 Mushroom Blend – *foursigmatic.com*

TROPICAL PRODUCE
Coconut – Whole Foods, *amazon.com*
Sapote – *amazon.com*
Cactus Pears – fresh in season from August to December in some Whole Foods markets
(for frozen unsweetened puree) – For the Gourmet *amazon.com*
(for sweetened puree) – *theperfectpuree.com*
Guavas (Goiaba) – *amafruits.com*
Dragon fruit – *pitayaplus.com*

SWEETNERS/STEVIA – *nunaturals.com*

PROBIOTICS – goodbelly.com. Whole Foods, *amazon.com*

PREBIOTICS – *msprebiotic.com, ora.organic.com*

BONE BROTH – *bonafideprovisions.com, butchersbonebroth.com, barebonebroth.com*

WATERS
Clean bottled water – *finewaters.com*
Coconut water – *harmlessharvest.com*
Cactus water – *drinkcaliwater.com*

SWIMWEAR – *dosgardenias.com*

ADDITIONAL RECIPES – *projectyoubewell.com*

FOOTNOTES

1. Robert D. Young, 'Validated Living Worldwide Supercentenarians', *Rejuvenation Research*. February 2017, 20(1): 64-66. Gerontology Research Group.

2. Buettner, Dan. *The Blue Zones*. Second ed. Washington DC.: National Geographic Partners, 2012. Print.

3. Willie Victor, Essentials for Health.

4. Kohn, David. 'Joint Pain, From the Gut', *The Atlantic*. Atlantic Media Company, 12 Jan. 2015. Web. 17 Mar. 2017.

5. Willie Victor, Essentials for Health.

6. *Happy Gut: The Cleansing Program to Help You Lose Weight, Gain Energy, and Eliminate Pain*. Vincent Pedre. William Morrow, 29 Dec. 2015, pp. 11-12.

7. *Happy Gut: The Cleansing Program to Help You Lose Weight, Gain Energy, and Eliminate Pain*. Vincent Pedre. William Morrow, 29 Dec. 2015, p. 19.

8. Campbell, Andrew W. 'Autoimmunity and the Gut' *Autoimmune Diseases*. Hindawi Publishing Corporation, 13 May 2014.

9. *Happy Gut*, Vincent Pedre, p 21.

10. Willie Victor, Essentials for Health.

11. Dr. Lisa Miller, ND, Deane Alban, 'Brain Fog: Causes, Symptoms and Solutions', *bebrainfit.com/stop-brain-fog-know-the-causes-symptoms-and-solutions*.

12. See *NRDC.org* for mercury levels in fish.

13. Willie Victor, Essentials for Health.

14. Lehman, Shereen, MS. 'Free Radicals in the Body', *Verywell*, Web. 20, July, 2016.

15. *phytochemicals.info/antioxidants.php*

16. Ravensthorpe, Michael. 'The Australian Kakadu Plum Is Rich in Vitamin C and Phytochemicals.' *NaturalNews*. Natural News, 6 June 2013.

17. Based on interview (September 2016) with Graham Firrell, owner Go Wild Australia.

18. Rowan, Claire. 'Interview: Truffles tap into the Omega-3 Benefits of Ahiflowers.' FoodBev Media. N.p., 31 Mar. 2016.

19. Cathy Wong, ND. 'Is Matcha Better for You Than Regular Green Tea?' *Verywell*. N.p., 31 Mar. 2016. Web. 22 Mar. 2017.

2O. Klein, Sarah. '6 Health Benefits Of Turmeric', *The Huffington Post*. 18 Oct. 2014.

21. *E3Live.com*

22. Information provided by Dr. Wayne Coates, researcher for Genesis Pure Mila chia seed. For more information go to *genesispure.com*.

23. McMillen, Matt. 'Mushrooms: What's Edible, Medicinal, and Psychedelic', *WebMD*.

24. Appleton, Nancy, PhD. 'Sugar's Health Effects, Risks & Problems: Is Sugar Sweet Poison?', *Healing Cancer Naturally*.

25. Heid, Markham. 'Does Bone Broth Really Have Health Benefits?', *Time*. Time, 6 Jan. 2016.

26. "Hearn, Nancy, 'Drinking Spring Water - Health Pros and Cons', *Water Benefits Health*, 2012.

27. Willie Victor, Essentials for Health.

28. Beddoe, A.F. *Biologic Ionization As Applied to Human Nutrition*. N.p.: Wendell Whitman, 2002.

29. Lefort N et al., Dietary Buglossoides Arvensis Oil Increases Circulating n-3 Polyunsaturated Fatty Acids in a Dose-Dependent Manner and Enhances Lipopolysaccharide-Stimulated Whole Blood Interleukin-10—A Randomized Placebo-Controlled Trial, Nutrients 2017, 9, 261; doi:10.3390/nu9030261.

30. Based on interview (September 2016) with Dr. Miller, ND.

31. Glassman, Keri. "Foods That Boost Collagen That Aren't Bone Broth." Nutritious Life, 4 Oct. 2017, *nutritiouslife.com/nurture-yourself/foods-that-boost-collagen*.

32. Dr. Jessica Wu, 'Eating For Beauty: The Best Diet For Healthy, Clear Skin', *Feed Your Face*; Sarah Wu, Forbes, September 14, 2014.

33. Anshul Gambhir, M.D., 'Vitamin C And Its Role In Skin Care', *drgambhir.com*.

34. Belleza Skincare Institute.

35. Fitzpatrick, T. B. (1975). 'Soleil et peau' [Sun and skin]. *Journal de Médecine Esthétique* (in French) (2): 33–34.

36. Allison Quistgard Scherer, medical aesthetician and owner of Sprig and Glow.

37. Cooney, Suzie. *How to Increase Your Stand Up Paddling Performance*. CreateSpace, 2015.

38. "Adler, Tamar, 'Breaking Point', Beauty & Fitness, *Vogue*, November, 2015: 178, 180.

39. Russell, Amanda. 'Over-Exercising or Simply Burned Out: The Seven Serious Signs', *The Huffington Post*. 20 June 2013.

40. To find a studio nearest you go to *thedaileymethod.com*.

41. Dr. Mercola, 'What Happens in Your Body When You're Sleep Deprived?', March 03, 2016.

42. Dr. Lisa Miller, ND.

43. Deepak Chopra, M.D. and David Simon, M.D. *Primordial Sound Meditation*. See *chopra.com*.

44. Deepak Chopra, M.D. and David Simon, M.D. *Primordial Sound Meditation*. See *chopra.com*.

45. Dr. James A. Coan, 'Social Regulation of the Neural Response to Threat Psychological Science', Dec 1, 2006; pp. 1032–1039.

46. Field, T.M., Sunshine, W., Hernandez-Reif, M., Quintino, O., Schanberg, S., Kuhn, C., & Burman, I. (1997). 'Massage therapy effects on depression and somatic symptoms in chronic fatigue syndrome', *Journal of Chronic Fatigue Syndrome*, 3, 43-51, *www6.miami.edu/touch-research*.

47. 'What Is Ayurvedic Massage?' Holistic And Ayurvedic Massage and Beauty Treatments in Rochester and Kent. Serenity Holistic Treatments.

Photos from Adobe Stock

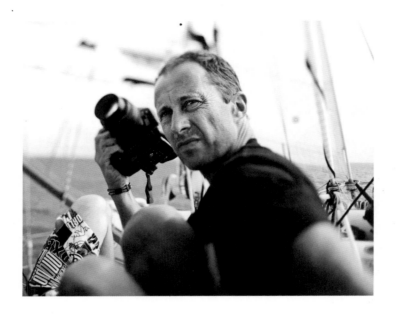

Born and raised in Paris, Franck Berthuot has been living and shooting in Hawaii for more than a decade. After a back injury while surfing, Franck naturally dove back into the water and began photographing athletes in the famous waves of Maui. Starting out as an action sports photographer, he soon became interested in capturing beautiful images of women in raw nature but focusing on the fashion aspect. His current body of work experiments with heavily contrasted black and white photography and explores working with additional lighting elements combined with outside natural lighting.

"I love the un-known underwater environment as well as capturing the beauty of people interacting with nature."

Visit Franck at www.frankiebees.com.

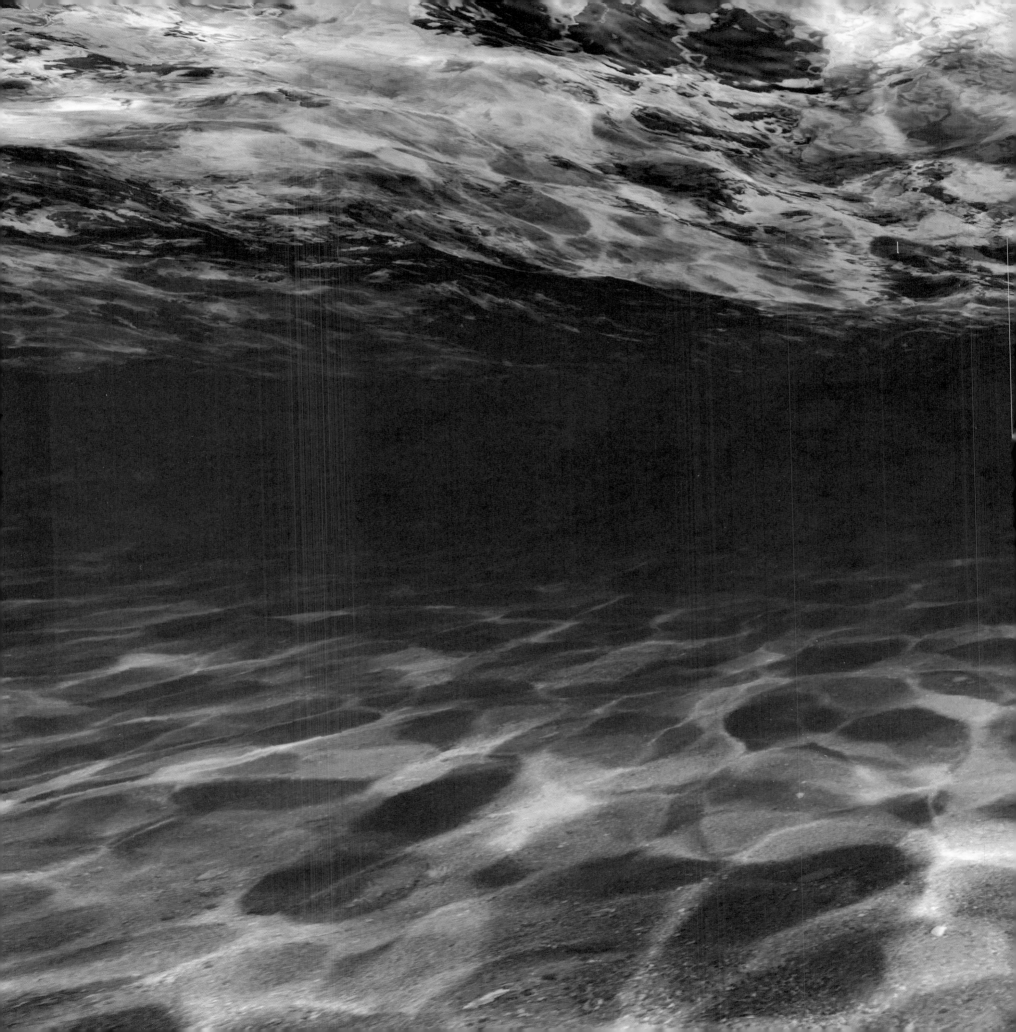